The Science of Pleasure

Exploring G-Spot and P-Spot Sensations

By
Dr. Sophia Hartman

The Science of Pleasure

Exploring G-Spot and P-Spot Sensations

Table of Contents

Introduction

Sexual pleasure is an integral aspect of human life, yet it's often shrouded in mystery, societal taboos, and personal inhibitions. This book is designed to shed light on the enigmatic yet immensely rewarding realms of G-Spot and P-Spot stimulation. Whether you're on a solo journey of self-discovery or looking to deepen the intimacy and pleasure in your relationship, the knowledge contained within these pages will serve as your trusted guide.

Our aim is to empower you with accurate, science-based information that will enable you to explore your body and your partner's body with confidence and curiosity. We'll delve deep into the anatomy, techniques, and psychological aspects that underpin meaningful and fulfilling intimate experiences. By providing a comprehensive understanding, you'll be equipped to navigate both the delights and challenges that may arise along the way.

The G-Spot and P-Spot have both been subjects of fascination and controversy over the years. Despite extensive studies and personal testimonials, myths and misconceptions still prevail. One of our first steps is to demystify these areas by presenting clear, evidence-based information. You'll find sections dedicated to the scientific research that informs our understanding, alongside practical techniques that can be applied immediately for enhanced pleasure.

But knowledge here isn't solely physical. Our exploration goes beyond mere anatomy. It encompasses the mind-body connection, emotional readiness, and the crucial aspect of communication between partners. Sexuality doesn't exist in a vacuum; it's influenced by our mental state, emotions, and the dynamics of our relationships. Therefore, understanding the psychological facets is as important as understanding the physical ones.

For those who engage in solo play, specific chapters will guide you step-by-step through techniques that enhance personal pleasure. Solo exploration is a vital aspect of sexual well-being, giving you the freedom to understand your body's responses outside the complexities of a partnership. This self-awareness can greatly enrich partnered experiences, making you more informed and confident in communicating your desires.

For couples, the dual exploration can be a profound journey of mutual discovery and connection. Understanding and practicing the techniques for G-Spot and P-Spot stimulation can open new doors to pleasure and deepen the emotional bonds between partners. We'll cover everything from the initial conversation about trying something new to advanced techniques that can take your intimate connection to unprecedented heights.

We also prioritize safety and hygiene, addressing common concerns and providing practical advice to ensure your experiences are as safe as they are pleasurable. These sections are essential reading, aimed at dispelling any worries that might otherwise hinder your exploration.

The art of sexual pleasure is a blend of the physical and the mental, the scientific and the emotional. As you journey through this book, you'll find that the destination isn't simply about achieving orgasm, but about enriching the entire spectrum of your sexual experiences. Each chapter is designed to build upon the last, gradually enhancing your understanding and capabilities in a way that feels both natural and exciting.

In the many pages that follow, you'll also encounter sections that address common challenges and offer ways to overcome them. Sexual exploration can sometimes bring about unexpected sensations or discomforts. It's crucial to approach these moments with patience and understanding, and our advice aims to help you navigate these experiences successfully.

We've dedicated specific chapters to combining G-Spot and clitoral stimulation, as well as P-Spot and penile stimulation. These combinations can offer blended orgasms and dual pleasures that amplify your sexual satisfaction. We'll guide you through these complex yet rewarding techniques with clear, step-by-step instructions.

A crucial aspect of our guide is the holistic approach to integrating these forms of stimulation into a healthy sex life. Sexual exploration doesn't have to be a separate endeavor; it should complement and enhance your overall sexual health and intimacy. We'll discuss ways to balance these practices within the context of a satisfying and vibrant sex life.

Finally, the book will close with an extensive glossary and a section for further reading and resources. These appendices are designed to provide you with additional avenues for exploration and learning, extending your journey beyond the confines of these pages.

So, whether you're a seasoned explorer of sexual terrains or taking your first steps into these uncharted waters, this book is crafted to support, educate, and inspire you. Let's embark on this journey together, discovering the profound joys that lie in the nuanced and deeply personal world of sexual pleasure.

Chapter 1:
Understanding Sexual Pleasure

Understanding sexual pleasure is an essential step toward a fulfilling and deeply intimate life. It's a multidimensional experience that weaves together the physical, emotional, and mental facets of our beings. From the electric tingle of anticipation to the soul-soothing warmth of connection, sexual pleasure is as much about our bodies responding to touch as it is about our minds engaging with sensations and emotions. The journey to unlocking deeper sexual pleasure often begins with self-awareness and open communication. As we delve into the intricate dance between the brain and the body, it's clear that the main ingredient isn't technique alone but the loving attention we bring to ourselves and our partners. By exploring the foundations of sexual pleasure and the pivotal role of the brain in sexual response, we tap into a reservoir of joy and connection that enriches our intimate experiences beyond measure.

Foundations of Sexual Pleasure

Sexual pleasure, while innately personal and subjective, is rooted in an intricate foundation of both physiological and psychological elements. Understanding these foundational aspects not only enhances individual experiences but also contributes to more fulfilling and intimate connections with partners. At its core, sexual pleasure is an amalgamation of physical sensations, emotional intimacy, and cognitive processes that together create deeply satisfying experiences.

Physiologically, the human body is equipped with a network of erogenous zones, nerve endings, and sensory receptors that respond to various stimuli. These areas are rich in nerve endings and can produce intense feelings of pleasure when stimulated. While some zones like the genitals are universally recognized, others such as the neck, ears, and inner thighs can be equally pleasurable. The responsiveness of these areas can vary greatly between individuals, highlighting the importance of personal exploration and communication with partners. This unique map of pleasure is a testament to the body's capacity for diverse and profound sexual experiences.

Now, let's turn our focus to the brain, the central hub of sexual pleasure. It's often said that the brain is the largest sex organ, and this couldn't be more accurate. Neural pathways and brain regions such as the hypothalamus and amygdala play critical roles in sexual arousal and orgasm. The brain interprets sensory inputs, triggers hormonal responses, and even influences emotional connections, creating a holistic sexual experience that transcends mere physical touch. Understanding these neural processes allows individuals to better harness and enhance their own sexual pleasure.

On an emotional level, sexual pleasure is deeply intertwined with feelings of intimacy, trust, and connection. Emotional safety and vulnerability can dramatically impact one's ability to experience pleasure. When individuals feel emotionally connected to their partners, they're more likely to engage fully and openly in sexual activities, leading to more gratifying experiences. The interplay of these emotions not only strengthens relationships but also enriches the quality of sexual encounters.

Moreover, the psychological aspect of sexual pleasure cannot be overlooked. Our thoughts, fantasies, and mental states significantly shape our sexual experiences. Stress, anxiety, and societal pressures often hinder sexual enjoyment, making it crucial to cultivate a healthy mental outlook. Mindfulness practices, positive self-talk, and cultivating a nonjudgmental attitude toward one's body and desires can profoundly boost sexual satisfaction. Embracing one's sexuality with confidence and openness lays a robust foundation for pleasurable and fulfilling experiences.

Cultural and societal influences also play a significant role in shaping perceptions and experiences of sexual pleasure. Societal norms, religious beliefs, and cultural taboos can either facilitate or hinder open exploration of sexuality. By challenging outdated norms and educating oneself about diverse perspectives on sexual pleasure, individuals can break free from restrictive mindsets and fully embrace their sexual potential. This shift not only fosters personal growth but also paves the way for more inclusive and respectful discourse around sex and pleasure.

A fundamental aspect of understanding sexual pleasure is acknowledging its dynamic and evolving nature. Sexual pleasure varies throughout one's life due to factors such as age, hormonal changes, and life experiences. Being aware of and adapting to these changes ensures that one's sexual well-being remains a priority. Engaging in continuous learning, seeking professional guidance when necessary, and maintaining open communication with partners can help navigate these shifts, ensuring sustained pleasure and intimacy over time.

John and Maria, a couple in their mid-thirties, discovered that their sexual pleasure significantly improved when they began prioritizing emotional intimacy and effective communication. They realized that by sharing their fantasies and desires openly, they could better understand and fulfill each other's needs. This practice not only enhanced their sexual experiences but also deepened their emotional connection, illustrating the profound impact of psychological and emotional factors on sexual pleasure.

The foundation of sexual pleasure isn't only about understanding the 'how' but also the 'why.' Delving into the reasons behind our sexual responses and desires fosters a more profound appreciation of our sexuality. When individuals recognize that pleasure is a holistic experience influenced by physical, emotional, and psychological factors, they become empowered to take control of their sexual health and well-being. This awareness encourages experimentation and openness to new experiences, ultimately leading to a richer and more satisfying sexual life.

In sum, the foundations of sexual pleasure are built upon a complex interplay of physiological, emotional, and psychological elements. By understanding and embracing these factors, individuals can enhance their sexual experiences, foster deeper connections with their partners, and cultivate a fulfilling and dynamic sexual life. As you continue to explore your own sexuality, remember that the journey itself is as important as the destination. By prioritizing self-awareness, open communication, and continual learning, you create the perfect conditions for a lifetime of pleasure and intimacy.

The Role of the Brain in Sexual Response

Understanding the complexities of sexual pleasure requires delving deep into the brain's involvement in sexual response. While the physical aspects of arousal often get the limelight, it's the brain that orchestrates, amplifies, and fine-tunes these sensations into a symphony of pleasure. This section explores how various brain regions and neurotransmitters contribute to sexual response, shaping our experiences in deeply personal and profound ways.

The brain plays a pivotal role in sexual arousal and pleasure by integrating sensory inputs with emotional and cognitive reactions. The journey of sexual arousal begins in the limbic system, a set of structures deep within the brain responsible for emotion and motivation. Key components include the hypothalamus, which regulates hormonal activity, and the amygdala, which processes emotions. Together, these areas help transform sensory stimuli into sexual excitement.

An essential aspect of sexual arousal is the release of neurotransmitters, the chemical messengers of the brain. Dopamine, often dubbed the "pleasure chemical," is released during sexual activity, creating feelings of euphoria and reward. It's the same chemical involved in other rewarding activities, like eating and socializing, which explains why sexual pleasure can feel so intensely gratifying. Other neurotransmitters, such as serotonin and oxytocin, also play significant roles. Serotonin can influence mood and emotional state, while oxytocin, known as the "cuddle hormone," fosters intimacy and bonding, especially post-orgasm.

The cortical areas of the brain are equally important in sexual response. The brain's largest part, the cerebral cortex, processes perceptions, thoughts, and memories. During sexual arousal, the prefrontal cortex, which is involved in complex thinking and decision-making, often becomes less active. This temporary dampening of activity helps us let go of inhibitions and immerse ourselves in the moment, enhancing our sexual experience.

Another fascinating aspect involves the brain's role in sexual fantasies and desires. The mental imagery and thoughts we engage in can significantly heighten arousal. The brain's visual and auditory cortexes help create vivid fantasies that complement the physical sensations of sexual activity. This mental engagement is critical for achieving a fully satisfying sexual experience, as it enables us to explore desires and scenarios that might not be feasible in real life.

Interestingly, research indicates that men and women might experience brain activity differences during sexual arousal. For instance, studies using brain imaging techniques reveal that women's brains often show increased activity in emotion-related regions compared to men. These differences underscore the nuanced ways in which the brain governs sexual response and highlight the importance of understanding individual variations.

The brain's involvement doesn't stop at arousal and orgasm; it plays a crucial role across the whole spectrum of sexual interactions. This includes the anticipation and build-up to sexual activity, which involves the reward pathways and enhances the desire to engage in sexual behavior. Furthermore, after sexual activity, the brain regulates the refractory period – a phase of reduced arousal following orgasm – which varies among individuals based on factors like age and health.

Mental health can also significantly impact sexual response. Conditions such as anxiety and depression can alter neurotransmitter levels and hormonal balance, leading to decreased sexual desire and performance. Similarly, psychological factors like stress and past traumas can affect the brain's ability to process sexual stimuli positively, emphasizing the deep connection between mental and sexual well-being.

Partner communication and emotional connection are other areas where the brain's role becomes evident. Effective communication about desires, boundaries, and fantasies can enhance intimacy and make the sexual experience more fulfilling. The brain processes these interactions, fostering a sense of security and bonding, thus improving overall sexual satisfaction. This interconnectedness between cognitive processes and emotional states underscores the importance of communication in building a healthy and pleasurable sexual relationship.

It's also important to address the impact of substances on sexual response. Alcohol and recreational drugs can significantly alter brain function, affecting neurotransmitter levels and impairing judgment, which can lead to risky sexual behaviors or a diminished sexual experience. Understanding how these substances interact with the brain can help individuals make informed choices about their use and its impact on their sexual health.

Neuroplasticity, the brain's ability to reorganize itself by forming new neural connections, plays a role in adapting to different sexual experiences over time. This ability is crucial for overcoming negative sexual experiences or trauma. By engaging in positive and enjoyable sexual activities, individuals can reshape their neural pathways, leading to improved sexual health and pleasure.

In conclusion, the brain is more than just a passenger in the journey of sexual pleasure; it's the conductor that shapes, enhances, and defines our sexual experiences. From neurotransmitter release to emotional processing and cognitive engagement, the brain's intricate network of functions ensures that sexual pleasure is a deeply enriching part of human experience. By understanding and appreciating the brain's role, individuals and couples can explore new dimensions of intimacy and pleasure, empowering themselves to create fulfilling sexual experiences.

Chapter 2:
Anatomy of the G-Spot

A s we venture into the intricate world of the G-Spot, we're diving into more than just physicality; we're exploring a realm of profound sensitivity and pleasure. Nestled within the anterior wall of the vagina, typically about one to three inches from the entrance, lies this remarkable area. It's not a distinct gland or organ, but rather a convergence of tissues, nerve endings, and glands – notably Skene's glands – that respond intensely to gentle pressure and rhythmic stimulation. Understanding the anatomy of the G-Spot is about grasping its potential to transform sexual experiences. By attuning to its unique sensitivities, one can unlock waves of pleasure that are both deeply fulfilling and intimately bonding. This chapter sets the stage for exploring the G-Spot's full potential, grounding our journey in anatomical clarity and empathetic explorations.

Locating the G-Spot

The G-Spot, a somewhat enigmatic feature of the human anatomy, has garnered fascination and curiosity over the years. Embarking on the journey to locate the G-Spot can be both an educational and pleasurable experience. A comprehensive understanding, coupled with exploration fueled by curiosity and care, can transform the intimate lives of individuals and couples.

First and foremost, it's essential to understand that the G-Spot is not a distinct, isolated organ but rather a network of tissues interconnected with various sensitive regions. Located on the anterior (front) wall of the vagina, the G-Spot generally resides about 1-3 inches inside, between the vaginal opening and the back of the pubic bone. Gently feeling for a textured area that might feel slightly different from the surrounding tissues can be your first clue. This area can become more prominent and sensitive with arousal and stimulation.

While anatomical textbooks might depict the human body in static terms, the G-Spot is dynamic. Its prominence and level of sensitivity can fluctuate based on factors such as arousal, emotional state, and individual variation. In some, the G-Spot may be more noticeable or sensitive than in others. It's important to approach this exploration without pressure, understanding that each person's experience is unique.

Communication plays a vital role in this exploration. Couples can enhance their connection by discussing their desires, boundaries, and preferences before engaging in any physical exploration. Establishing a comfortable and consensual environment is crucial. For solo explorers, being in a relaxed state of mind and allowing oneself to be present in the moment can lead to more fulfilling discoveries.

When starting the journey to locate the G-Spot, ensure that both the mind and body are sufficiently aroused and relaxed. This state of arousal can be achieved through foreplay, engaging the senses through touch, sound, or even aromatherapy. Once a sense of comfort and anticipation is established, begin the physical exploration.

Use a well-lubricated finger (or fingers) to gently explore the vaginal canal. Follow the natural curve of the front wall. Many find a "come hither" motion—using one or two fingers curved towards the belly button—to be particularly effective in stimulating the G-Spot. This motion not only helps in locating the textured area but also increases arousal.

Some might find it beneficial to experiment with various angles and pressures. Applying steady, rhythmic pressure can create a buildup of sensation. Once you locate the area that feels distinct, continue to explore with varying motions and pressures to understand what feels most pleasurable. Remember, patience and gentle persistence are key.

It's worth noting that the G-Spot is part of a larger erogenous network and its sensations are interconnected with clitoral and vaginal stimuli. The sensations triggered by G-Spot stimulation can range from gentle pleasure to intense, full-body orgasms. However, it's essential to approach this with an open mind, free from expectations of immediate results or specific types of pleasure.

In the initial stages of exploration, some individuals might not find the G-Spot right away. This is completely normal. The journey to understand and connect with your own body or your partner's body is ongoing. Revisiting this exploration with varying levels of arousal and different techniques can yield new discoveries over time.

Partners can play a significant role by observing and responding to non-verbal cues. Changes in breathing, vocal expressions of pleasure, and subtle body movements can guide where to focus and how to adjust the stimulation. This shared experience can deepen the emotional and physical bond between partners.

Exploring the G-Spot isn't just an act; it's a dance of intimacy and curiosity. Each touch, each sensation, is a step towards a more profound understanding of bodily pleasure. This nuanced approach to exploring the G-Spot can redefine personal and shared sexual experiences, elevating them from routine to revelatory.

The empowerment that comes from understanding one's own body or a partner's body cannot be overstated. Knowing where the G-Spot is and how it responds can bring a sense of control and confidence in intimate settings. It encourages deeper conversations about desires and boundaries, fostering a healthy and enriching sexual relationship.

Moreover, this exploration isn't reserved for the young and adventurous alone. People of all ages can benefit from understanding the G-Spot. It's never too late to deepen your knowledge and enhance your intimate experiences. The G-Spot holds potential for pleasure and connection that transcends age.

In conclusion, locating the G-Spot is not just about finding a physical spot. It's about embracing the journey of discovery, understanding, and connection. Whether you're exploring solo or with a partner, approach this exploration with open-hearted curiosity, patience, and communication. The rewards are not merely physical but encompass emotional intimacy and personal empowerment.

Structures and Sensitivities

Understanding the structures and sensitivities of the G-spot can be a gateway to unlocking layers of pleasure. The G-spot, or Gräfenberg spot, is more than just a single entity; it's a network intricately connected to a variety of tissues and nerves. Delving into this complexity requires a mix of scientific curiosity and the willingness to explore personal experiences. Let's begin by unpacking the anatomy.

Firstly, the G-spot is located on the anterior wall of the vagina, a few inches in. This area is supported by a rich network of sensitive tissues. It involves periurethral glands, ducts, and the deeper layers of the clitoral network, all of which converge to form the notorious spot. It's this mixture of anatomical structures that contributes to the sometimes elusive nature of G-spot stimulation.

The periurethral glands, often compared to the male prostate, play a pivotal role. When stimulated, these glands can lead to enhanced sexual arousal and might even produce a fluid. This is part of why some people experience female ejaculation or "squirting" — though it's a topic mired in both fascination and debate.

Equally significant is the clitoral network, which extends far beyond the external button most think of as the clitoris. The internal clitoris has extensive branches that wrap around the vaginal walls, intertwining with the tissues that form the G-spot. Thus, G-spot stimulation can indirectly involve the clitoris, amplifying the overall experience.

What makes this area distinctive is its sensitivity. The skin and tissues forming the G-spot are densely packed with nerve endings. These nerve endings make it responsive to different kinds of touch — from gentle caresses to more vigorous stimuli. Understanding this can help tailor the experience to individual preferences.

The arousal of the G-spot follows a journey from subtle tingling to intense pleasure. When blood flow increases during sexual arousal, the G-spot becomes swollen, making it more prominent and easier to locate. It's like the body's way of guiding you towards hidden treasures of bliss.

This zone's sensitivity is by no means uniform. It's quite dynamic, reacting variably based on factors such as hormonal changes, arousal levels, and even emotional states. For some, initial pressures might feel uncomfortable, while for others it could be immediately pleasurable. Listening to the body's cues and adjusting accordingly is key.

Interestingly, the G-spot's sensitivity is also influenced by the surrounding pelvic floor muscles. These muscles play a role in sexual function, and their tone can impact how one experiences G-spot stimulation. Strengthening these muscles through exercises like Kegels can sometimes heighten sensations.

Beyond physical structures, there's an emotional component that can't be ignored. The psychological state can greatly affect how the G-spot responds to touch. Feeling relaxed, connected, and in tune with your partner — or yourself — can greatly enhance the experience.

As we delve deeper into its complexities, it's essential to remember that every individual's anatomy and sensitivity levels are unique. What works for one person might not work for another, and that's perfectly normal. Embracing this uniqueness can transform the journey into an explorative adventure.

To truly harness the potential of the G-spot, it's valuable to combine anatomical knowledge with communication. Whether it's a solo exploration or shared with a partner, discussing feelings, preferences, and boundaries can help create a more fulfilling experience. Open conversations about desires and sensations foster mutual understanding and can guide better, more tailored approaches.

Wrap all this in a blend of curiosity and patience, and the exploration of the G-spot can become a deeply enriching journey. This knowledge forms the foundation for advanced techniques and mindful practices that aim to amplify intimate experiences, building a more confident approach to sexual pleasure.

In summary, the G-spot is a symphony of anatomical structures and sensitivities that react dynamically to different stimuli. By understanding its complexity and embracing individual differences, the journey toward discovering and enjoying the G-spot can be a rewarding and deeply satisfying experience.

Chapter 3:
Anatomy of the P-Spot

The P-Spot, or prostate gland, is an often-overlooked powerhouse of male pleasure. Nestled just a few inches inside the rectum, this walnut-sized organ is responsible for producing seminal fluid and plays a crucial role in sexual arousal and orgasm. Its unique sensitivity can open new doors of ecstasy for those willing to explore its full potential. Understanding the anatomy of the P-Spot is essential: it essentially encompasses the anterior surface of the rectum, directly beneath the bladder, making it accessible and highly responsive to gentle stimulation. When aroused, the P-Spot can elicit profoundly pleasurable sensations, often described as a deep, fulfilling pulse of pleasure that radiates throughout the body. This chapter aims to guide you through the intricacies of locating and understanding this integral part of the male anatomy, offering you and your partner an opportunity to experience elevated intimacy and gratification through scientifically-informed techniques.

Finding the P-Spot

Embarking on the journey of discovering the P-Spot can be both exciting and transformative. Rooted deep within male anatomy, the P-Spot—more commonly known as the prostate gland—holds the potential for immense pleasure and even profound emotional experiences. Often misunderstood or overlooked, understanding how to locate the P-Spot is the foundational step in unlocking its full pleasure potential.

The first thing to recognize about the P-Spot is its anatomical location. The prostate gland is situated just below the bladder and in front of the rectum. This walnut-sized organ is part of the male reproductive system and is often described as having a slightly spongy texture. It's not visible externally, which is why tactile exploration is crucial.

To find the P-Spot, start by ensuring that both you and your partner are comfortable and relaxed. This is essential because tension can make the process uncomfortable. Gently massaging the perineum—the area between the scrotum and the anus—can help loosen the muscles and prepare you for the experience. This area is rich in nerve endings and acts as a good starting point for stimulation.

Once relaxed, the next step is to introduce a lubricated finger or a specially designed prostate massager into the rectum. Quality lubrication cannot be overstated; it reduces friction and makes the experience more enjoyable. Slowly and gently, insert the finger or massager about 2-3 inches into the rectum, curving it towards the front of the body. The P-Spot is located on the anterior wall of the rectum, about one to two inches in. You'll know you've found it when you feel a slightly raised, smooth area that is somewhat firmer than the surrounding tissue.

Initial sensations might vary, ranging from mild to intensely pleasurable. A light, rhythmic motion—akin to the "come hither" gesture—can help in identifying the sweet spot. Unlike other forms of stimulation, the P-Spot might require a bit more patience initially, as it adapts to this new kind of touch. As you continue to explore, communicate openly about what feels good, adjusting pressure and movement as needed.

Sensory exploration is highly individual, so don't be discouraged if the eureka moment isn't immediate. Some may experience initial sensations as strange or even uncomfortable, but with practice and patience, these can evolve into deeply pleasurable experiences. Differing from penile stimulation, the gratification derived from P-Spot stimulation can feel more profound, spreading warmth throughout the pelvic region and sometimes leading to full-body orgasms.

For many, P-Spot exploration is also a pathway to expanding emotional intimacy. The vulnerability involved in this kind of exploration can foster trust and deepen the connection between partners. Talk openly about boundaries and comfort levels, ensuring that both parties are enthusiastic about the experience.

Integrating P-Spot stimulation into your intimate routine can significantly enhance sexual satisfaction. Varied touch and changing patterns of movement can unveil different types of pleasure. Avoid repetitive actions; instead, experiment with alternating between gentle circling motions and firmer pressure to see how the sensations evolve.

Pay attention to feedback from your body or your partner's body. Notice muscle contractions, changes in breathing, and verbal or physical cues. These signs can guide you towards more pleasurable techniques.

Practice mindfulness. Being present in the moment can amplify the sensations and the overall experience.

As you delve deeper into the practice, you may discover that P-Spot orgasms bring about a different kind of release. These orgasms can be less intense but more prolonged than penile orgasms, offering an entirely new dimension of pleasure. For those who experience both types, combining them can lead to incredibly powerful and fulfilling encounters.

Additionally, the health benefits of P-Spot stimulation contribute to its appeal. Regular prostate massages can help improve circulation and may reduce the risk of prostate issues later in life. This merging of pleasure and health makes finding the P-Spot not just an exploration of joy, but an investment in long-term well-being.

Embrace the adventure of finding and stimulating the P-Spot. Every body is unique, and what works wonders for one person might not be the golden standard for another. The key lies in exploration, patience, and an open mind. Accept the journey with curiosity and a willingness to discover new realms of pleasure and intimacy.

Remember, the P-Spot is not just an anatomical feature; it is a gateway to deeper connections, emotional intimacy, and enhanced physical pleasure. Whether you are exploring solo or with a partner, the journey to discovering the P-Spot can be one of the most rewarding aspects of your sexual experience. Let this guide pave the way for you to uncover new dimensions of enjoyment and connection, transcending the ordinary to reach truly extraordinary experiences.

Male Prostate Anatomy

The male prostate, often referred to as the P-Spot, is a walnut-sized gland situated just below the bladder and in front of the rectum. Its role extends beyond mere reproductive functionality; it's integral to male sexual pleasure due to its rich nerve supply. Let's delve into this often misunderstood yet fascinating aspect of male anatomy.

Firstly, the prostate is composed of both glandular and muscular tissue. The glandular portion contributes to the production of seminal fluid, which nourishes and transports sperm during ejaculation. On the other hand, the muscular tissue helps with the expulsion of semen during orgasm. These dual functions highlight the prostate's crucial role in sexual and reproductive health.

From a practical standpoint, the prostate can be accessed and stimulated through the anterior wall of the rectum. This position makes it ideal for direct massage, which can evoke profound sensations and lead to prostate orgasms. It's essential to understand the proper techniques and approach to exploring the P-Spot safely and pleasurably, which we'll elaborate on in later chapters.

Notably, the prostate is surrounded by a plexus of nerves, commonly known as the prostatic nerve plexus. These nerves are responsible for its heightened sensitivity. When effectively stimulated, either through direct pressure or rhythmic motion, the prostate can produce intense waves of pleasure, often described as different from penile orgasms but equally, if not more, powerful.

This sensitivity also means that gentle and informed exploration is necessary. The prostate can be prone to discomfort if not approached with care. A good rule of thumb is to use ample lubrication and go slowly, paying close attention to the body's signals. It's also crucial to communicate openly with one's partner to ensure comfort and mutual enjoyment.

The physical structure of the prostate is divided into zones: the central zone, peripheral zone, transitional zone, and the anterior fibro-muscular stroma. The peripheral zone is most often associated with prostate cancer, while the transitional zone is usually the site of benign prostatic hyperplasia (BPH). For the purposes of pleasure, the focus tends to be on stimulating the entire gland rather than specific zones.

It's worth mentioning that the health of the prostate is integral to overall wellbeing. Conditions such as prostatitis, BPH, and prostate cancer can affect both sexual function and quality of life. Regular check-ups and awareness are key to maintaining prostate health, which will in turn support sexual pleasure. We'll cover safety and hygiene practices in greater detail in Chapter 17.

The male prostate is not just an anatomical structure but a source of immense pleasure. When approached with the right mindset and techniques, it can enhance intimacy and deepen connections between partners. Understanding its anatomy is the first step towards unlocking these possibilities.

In addition to its role in sexual pleasure, the prostate also has significant functions in urinary health. It encircles the urethra, the tube through which urine exits the body. This positioning means that any issues with the prostate, such as inflammation or enlargement, can lead to urinary symptoms. It's another reason why maintaining prostate health is paramount.

One fascinating aspect of prostate stimulation is the potential for multiple orgasms. Unlike penile orgasms, which often have a refractory period (a recovery phase where repeated arousal is difficult), prostate orgasms can be achieved sequentially. This opens up new realms of sexual experience and satisfaction, allowing for prolonged pleasure sessions.

The pursuit of understanding and embracing prostate pleasure is not just for those in committed relationships. Solo exploration can be an empowering journey of self-discovery, leading to better sexual health and an enhanced understanding of one's own body. Techniques for solo practice will be thoroughly explored in Chapter 11.

Throughout history, male prostate pleasure has been shrouded in misconceptions and stigma. However, contemporary sexuality educators and researchers are breaking down these barriers, leading to a more informed and liberated approach to male sexual health. By appreciating the anatomical and functional nuances of the prostate, individuals can enrich their sexual experiences and foster a deeper connection with their bodies.

In summary, the prostate, with its dual roles in reproduction and pleasure, is a pivotal part of male anatomy. Its sensitivity, when tapped into with care and knowledge, offers unique and profound pleasures. Understanding its structure and functions is crucial for those looking to explore the full spectrum of their sexual potential, alone or with a partner. As we continue through this book, we'll delve deeper into the techniques and practices that can help maximize prostate stimulation, ensuring a safe and fulfilling exploration of the P-Spot.

Chapter 4:
Scientific Research on the G-Spot

Through decades of research, the G-Spot has emerged from a whispered myth to an intriguing focal point for scientists and sexual health experts. This cluster of sensitive tissues, first popularized by Dr. Ernst Gräfenberg, has since been the subject of numerous studies that aim to understand its anatomical and functional significance. Advanced imaging techniques have allowed researchers to map the G-Spot's precise location and its connectivity within the broader network of sexual response. Contrary to earlier debates doubting its existence, most contemporary studies support that the G-Spot, while varying in sensitivity among individuals, is a legitimate source of sexual pleasure. By debunking myths and grounding their findings in empirical evidence, scientists aim to transform how we perceive and embrace G-Spot stimulation, fostering a more informed and liberated approach to sexual wellness.

Studies and Findings

Scientific curiosity about the G-Spot dates back several decades, driven by the desire to understand the intricacies of female sexual pleasure. One of the earliest modern studies, conducted in the 1980s by Dr. Ernst Gräfenberg—the individual for whom the G-Spot is named—marked a turning point in our understanding of this elusive area. Gräfenberg's work, while initially met with skepticism, laid the groundwork for more focused investigations into female sexual anatomy and response.

Since then, numerous studies have attempted to both confirm and delineate the existence and characteristics of the G-Spot. Some research efforts have employed anatomical investigations, while others have utilized self-reported data from individuals to gain a broader understanding. As a result, we now have a rich tapestry of findings that highlight both the complexity and subjectivity of sexual pleasure.

A study published in the "Journal of Sexual Medicine" utilized ultrasound technology to explore the anatomical differences in women's pelvic regions. Researchers identified a cluster of tissues along the vaginal wall that showed heightened sensitivity and, for some participants, was associated with intense pleasure when stimulated. This region, often described in relation to the urethral sponge, seems to serve as a focal point for sensations that many might describe as originating from the G-Spot.

Another pivotal study, led by Dr. Beverly Whipple and her colleagues, expanded on Gräfenberg's findings by introducing a more qualitative approach. They gathered self-reported experiences from women who had identified their own G-Spots and documented their responses to various stimulation techniques. This work underscored the variability in individual experiences and suggested that orgasmic response from G-Spot stimulation is highly personal and can be influenced by numerous factors, including emotional and psychological states.

Functional Magnetic Resonance Imaging (fMRI) has also been employed in more recent studies to observe brain activity in response to G-Spot stimulation. By capturing real-time brain images, researchers have been able to pinpoint areas of the brain that light up during sexual arousal and orgasm. These studies support the notion that the G-Spot isn't just an anatomical curiosity but is deeply connected to the brain's pleasure and reward systems.

In terms of biochemical responses, studies reveal that G-Spot stimulation often leads to a notable release of oxytocin—a hormone commonly associated with bonding and intimacy. This hormone surge can contribute to the overall intensity of the orgasmic experience and further illustrates the interconnectedness of physical and emotional aspects of sexual pleasure.

However, not all studies have reached the same conclusions. Some research has called into question the very existence of a distinct "G-Spot," arguing that the sensations reported might be attributable to other anatomical structures like the clitoral network. The clitoris, with its extensive internal structure, may overlap and interact with other sensitive areas, including what has traditionally been labeled the G-Spot.

This set of findings has led some researchers to suggest a re-framing of our understanding. Rather than viewing the G-Spot as a single, easily identifiable entity, it might be more accurate to consider it part of a broader "clitourethrovaginal complex." This perspective helps to encapsulate the intricate interplay of different structures within the female pelvis, each contributing to the sensation and pleasure that individuals can experience.

Interestingly, the quest for understanding the G-Spot has also involved cross-cultural studies. Research comparing concepts of female sexual pleasure across different societies has shown intriguing variations. In some cultures, descriptions of pleasure zones align closely with the concept of the G-Spot, while in others, this area is either less emphasized or viewed through a different lens entirely, reflecting diverse socio-cultural influences on sexual education and perception.

Given these nuances, a meta-analysis of existing literature on the G-Spot highlights the recurrent theme of individual variability. The findings collectively affirm that while the G-Spot might not be universally experienced in the same way by all women, it certainly plays a significant role in the sexual pleasure of many. This reinforces the importance of personalized approaches and open communication between partners when exploring G-Spot stimulation.

Data from surveys and focus groups further illustrate the diversity of experiences. Some women describe G-Spot orgasms as more intense and emotionally profound compared to clitoral orgasms, while others report no distinct difference. This variability emphasizes the subjective nature of sexual pleasure and the importance of mutual exploration and consent in intimate relationships.

The academic dialogue on this topic has prompted a broader conversation about the importance of female sexual health and empowerment. Studies consistently advocate for more comprehensive sexual education that includes detailed information about the G-Spot and other erogenous zones. This educational approach can empower individuals to better understand their own bodies and communicate more effectively with partners, thus enhancing their sexual well-being.

Despite the breadth of studies conducted, there remains much to discover. Ongoing research is continuously refining our understanding, particularly as advances in technology and methodology emerge. Scientists and sexologists continue to push boundaries, exploring new dimensions of the G-Spot and its role in overall sexual health. These efforts are not merely academic; they have real-world implications for enhancing the intimate lives of individuals and couples.

In conclusion, the scientific exploration of the G-Spot has provided valuable insights into the complexities of female sexual pleasure. While not without controversy or debate, the collective body of research underscores the significance of this area for many women. As scientific tools become more sophisticated and societal attitudes towards female sexuality grow more open and inclusive, we can look forward to even deeper understanding and appreciation of this remarkable aspect of human anatomy.

Ultimately, the quest to understand the G-Spot is a testament to the broader human journey towards deeper intimacy and connection. By staying informed and open to new discoveries, we can continue to foster healthier and more fulfilling sexual relationships, celebrating the intricate beauty of human sexuality in all its forms.

Debunking Myths

When it comes to the G-Spot, there are more than a few myths floating around that can easily mislead and misinform. One of the most persistent myths is the very existence of the G-Spot itself. Some argue that it's a figment of imagination, a mythical zone created to amplify sexual mystique. However, scientific research suggests otherwise. While the G-Spot might not be a distinct anatomical entity, it is a sensitive area that can yield immense pleasure when stimulated properly, often linked with the urethral sponge and other adjacent structures.

Another myth that needs debunking is that the G-Spot guarantees an orgasm. This isn't true for everyone. Just as some women may not experience orgasm through clitoral stimulation alone, the same can be said for G-Spot stimulation. The human body is wonderfully complex, and sexual pleasure can vary significantly from one person to another. It's critical to understand that there's no 'one-size-fits-all' when it comes to this. Listening to one's own body, experimenting with different techniques, and communicating with a partner are essential.

The myth that G-Spot orgasms are more intense than clitoral orgasms has also gained traction over the years. Objective measures of orgasm intensity are subjective at best. Some women report that G-Spot orgasms are deeper or more fulfilling, while others find clitoral orgasms just as powerful, if not more so. Each woman's experience is unique. The key takeaway should be that different types of stimulation can lead to different kinds of pleasurable experiences, none inherently superior to another.

A particularly damaging myth is that those who don't experience G-Spot pleasure are somehow 'missing out' or 'incomplete'. This couldn't be further from the truth. The pursuit of sexual pleasure should be about discovering what feels good for you or your partner, not about ticking off a list of supposed milestones. Focusing too much on the G-Spot can deprive individuals of discovering other equally satisfying erogenous zones.

Another pervasive myth involves the supposed difficulty of locating the G-Spot. While it can take some time and patience to find and stimulate, it is by no means an impossible task. Armed with correct knowledge and a willingness to explore, many have successfully discovered this sensitive area. Anatomical variations exist, making each individual's experience different. Simple techniques such as using a curved finger or specific sex toys designed for G-Spot stimulation can make the search less daunting.

The myth confusing urinary incontinence with squirting (or female ejaculation) also requires clarification. They are not the same. Squirting involves the expulsion of fluid from the paraurethral glands, which some scientists believe to be analogous to the male prostate. This natural process differs entirely from urinary incontinence, and understanding this can alleviate unnecessary stigma and embarrassment.

Moreover, there's a misconception that G-Spot stimulation should be painful or uncomfortable. If it is, you're probably doing it wrong or your body may not be aroused enough for this type of touch. The area should be approached gently and arousal should be enough to ensure comfort. Communication with your partner during this process is critical. Experimenting with different pressures and angles can lead to more pleasurable experiences without discomfort.

Many also believe only women with a certain anatomy can experience G-Spot pleasure. This is false. The variability in sensitivity and pleasure patterns doesn't correlate to a 'one-size' anatomical structure. This thinking excludes a broad spectrum of experiences and reinforces unnecessary limitations. Whether someone enjoys G-Spot stimulation or not can be influenced by many factors beyond just anatomy, such as emotional state, level of arousal, and previous sexual experiences.

There's also the myth that G-Spot stimulation is just for young, sexually active women. Sexual pleasure has no age limit, and the ability to experience G-Spot stimulation doesn't diminish with age. Indeed, many older women find that they become more comfortable and in tune with their bodies as they age, allowing them to explore and enjoy G-Spot stimulation in ways they might not have when they were younger.

Unfortunately, some myths can lead people to think that G-Spot stimulation requires expensive gadgets or specialist tools. While sex toys designed for G-Spot stimulation can enhance the experience, they're by no means necessary. Simple techniques using fingers can provide ample stimulation. Toys are an option, not a necessity, for those who wish to add variety.

Finally, there is the myth that the G-Spot is just a tool for achieving spectacular orgasms in heterosexual sex, often sidelining the experiences of LGBTQ+ individuals. However, sexual pleasure knows no orientation. Understanding and exploring the G-Spot can be just as enriching for lesbian, bisexual, and queer women as for their heterosexual counterparts. The principles that make G-Spot stimulation pleasurable are universal, transcending sexual orientation.

Debunking these myths is crucial for fostering a healthy, informed understanding of sexual pleasure. Breaking free from these misconceptions allows individuals and couples to approach intimacy with a sense of curiosity rather than fear or frustration. By dispelling these legends and focusing on what genuine scientific research tells us, we open the door to more satisfying and empowering sexual experiences. Remember, the journey to discovering the G-Spot and all its potentials is deeply personal. So, embrace it with openness and enthusiasm.

Chapter 5:
Scientific Research on the P-Spot

Scientific exploration into the P-Spot, or prostate, has surged in recent years, shedding light on an often overlooked avenue of male pleasure. Studies have revealed that stimulating the P-Spot can lead to intense orgasms and profound sexual satisfaction, much like the G-Spot in women. Key findings emphasize its role in enhancing sexual experiences, as well as promoting overall prostate health. This chapter dives deep into the seminal research that has demystified the P-Spot, dispelling outdated misconceptions and offering a science-backed perspective. With modern advancements, scientists and sexologists have mapped out its anatomical intricacies, demonstrating its potential not just for pleasure but also for intimate connection. Embracing this knowledge can empower individuals and couples to explore new dimensions of their sexual repertoire, leading to richer, more fulfilling experiences.

Key Scientific Discoveries

Scientific research on the P-Spot, also known as the prostate, has surged over the last few decades. One of the most enlightening discoveries is its role in male sexual pleasure. Although previously underappreciated, the prostate's importance has gained recognition, transforming how we understand male sexuality. Early studies thoroughly mapped out the anatomy of the P-Spot, revealing its proximity to the rectal wall and its sensitivity to stimulation.

One of the groundbreaking studies led by Dr. Beverly Whipple in the 1980s shed light on the P-Spot's potential for inducing orgasm. This research showed that when the prostate is stimulated correctly, it can elicit intense orgasms, sometimes described as more full-bodied than penile-driven orgasms. This expanded understanding has validated the experiences of countless men and opened the door for more inclusive discussions about male sexual health.

More recent studies have examined the biochemical processes triggered by P-Spot stimulation. Researchers found that prostate stimulation can lead to increased production of oxytocin and dopamine. These hormones are associated not only with pleasure but also with bonding and emotional intimacy. When understood in this light, the P-Spot is not just about physical gratification but can be a gateway to deeper emotional connections.

Another significant finding involves the role of the P-Spot in overall prostate health. Some studies suggest that regular prostate massage can reduce symptoms of benign prostatic hyperplasia (BPH) and prostatitis. This gives an added layer of importance to understanding and exploring the P-Spot, as it blends pleasure with potential health benefits, making it a topic of considerable interest for medical professionals as well.

The development of new tools and devices has also driven scientific discoveries. Innovations like prostate massagers and specialized toys have allowed researchers to explore various methods of stimulation and their effects on the body. These advances have facilitated greater self-exploration and partner play, yielding valuable insights into optimizing technique and comfort.

Furthermore, the diversity of the male sexual experience has been a focal point in recent research. Studies emphasize that not every man will experience P-Spot pleasure in the same way. Factors like anatomy and psychological preparedness can significantly influence the experience. As a result, personalized approaches to exploring the P-Spot have been encouraged, promoting a more inclusive and comprehensive understanding of male sexuality.

Research has also tackled the psychological barriers and societal stigmas surrounding P-Spot stimulation. The notion that prostate exploration is relegated solely to the realm of medical necessity or a niche sexual practice is steadily being debunked. By framing it as a natural and healthy part of male sexuality, more men feel empowered to explore this area without fear of judgment or self-doubt.

Clinical trials and anecdotal reports have added layers of credibility to the scientific discourse. For example, studies involving MRI scans have shown the neurological responses triggered by prostate stimulation, further supporting the physical and psychological benefits attributed to P-Spot play.

Integration of P-Spot research into broader sex education curricula has also been a critical scientific milestone. Teaching about the P-Spot in a normalized context helps remove taboos and encourages informed exploration. This integration ensures that future generations grow up with a more holistic understanding of their bodies and potential pleasure points.

Importantly, the role of education and open dialogue cannot be understated. Doctors, sex educators, and therapists have all played a part in disseminating information gleaned from scientific studies. Workshops, webinars, and literature on P-Spot stimulation have become more widely available, fostering a culture of curiosity and learning.

One potent area of ongoing research involves the potential therapeutic uses of P-Spot stimulation. Some studies are investigating how prostate massage can affect mood disorders and stress levels. By triggering the release of feel-good hormones, prostate stimulation could offer a supplementary approach to mental health treatments.

In summary, the key scientific discoveries surrounding the P-Spot have revolutionized our understanding of male pleasure and health. These advancements emphasize that the P-Spot is not merely an anatomical curiosity but a multifaceted part of male sexuality with far-reaching implications for pleasure, intimacy, and overall wellbeing. Such insights empower men to embrace a broader spectrum of sexual experiences, encouraging a more fulfilling and informed approach to intimacy.

Common Misconceptions

Scientific research on the P-Spot, also known as the prostate, is a field that continues to evolve, yet numerous misconceptions persist. One prevailing myth is that P-Spot stimulation is solely for homosexual men. This couldn't be further from the truth. The prostate is an anatomical feature of male biology, irrespective of one's sexual orientation. It is a source of pleasure that can be explored and enjoyed by anyone with a prostate, including heterosexual men.

This misconception holds back many from exploring what could be a deeply enriching part of their sexual lives. The social stigma surrounding P-Spot stimulation often stems from outdated views on masculinity and sexuality. These beliefs are perpetuated by a lack of education and open dialogue about male sexual health. The fact is, understanding and stimulating the P-Spot can open new avenues of pleasure and intimacy for many men and their partners.

Another common misconception is that P-Spot stimulation is inherently painful or uncomfortable. This fear can be a significant barrier to exploration. While it is true that the prostate is an internal structure accessed through the rectum, discomfort largely depends on technique and relaxation. Using adequate lubrication, communicating with a partner, and proceeding slowly can make the experience not only comfortable but highly enjoyable.

It is crucial to note that the discomfort often associated with prostate play comes from inadequate preparation or the use of inappropriate techniques. For example, using objects that are not designed for prostate stimulation or failing to relax the muscles in the area can lead to an unpleasant experience. On the other hand, when approaches are informed and considerate, the results can be remarkably satisfying.

Another misconception is that all men will experience the same level of pleasure from P-Spot stimulation. Human bodies are unique, and what works wonders for one person might not be as effective for another. Some men might find the sensation overwhelming in a pleasurable way, while others could be more neutral about it. It's important to approach P-Spot exploration with an open mind and realistic expectations.

Exploring the P-Spot should be seen as a journey rather than a destination. Achieving ejaculation through P-Spot stimulation is not the only measure of success. For many, the process of exploration can be as rewarding as the end result. The goal should focus on understanding one's own body and finding out what brings joy and satisfaction.

Another commonly held myth is that frequent P-Spot stimulation can lead to prostate issues or increase the risk of prostate cancer. Current scientific evidence does not support this claim. In fact, some studies suggest that regular ejaculation, whether through prostate stimulation or other means, may actually reduce the risk of prostate cancer. The key is to engage in these activities safely and hygienically to maintain good health.

Further, some people believe that achieving prostate orgasm is easy and straightforward. While some might experience immediate and intense pleasure, it often takes time and practice for others. Patience and persistence are essential. Like any skill, learning how to stimulate the P-Spot effectively can require some trial and error.

One more common misconception concerns the use of toys for P-Spot stimulation. Some individuals think that these toys are unsafe or that using them means something negative about their sexuality. In reality, toys designed for prostate stimulation can enhance the experience by providing the precise pressure and angles needed to stimulate the P-Spot effectively. It's vital to choose high-quality, body-safe materials to ensure both enjoyment and safety.

In addition, there is a belief that P-Spot stimulation can interfere with urinary function. While the prostate is part of the male urinary system, gentle and correct stimulation should not affect urination. In fact, some men report improved urinary health from regular prostate massages, as it can help reduce the tension and improve blood flow in the area.

Despite these misconceptions, the scientific community continues to uncover the complexities and potential of the P-Spot. Research demonstrates that stimulating the P-Spot can lead to intense pleasure, sometimes resulting in what is described as a "prostate orgasm." This type of orgasm can differ significantly from penile-induced orgasms, often being more intense and involving different sensations.

In summary, the misconceptions surrounding P-Spot stimulation are numerous and varied, often deeply rooted in social stigmas and misinformation. By educating ourselves and embracing open dialogue, we can challenge these myths and unlock new realms of pleasure and intimacy. Breaking free from these misconceptions allows individuals and couples to explore their sexuality more fully and with greater confidence.

Chapter 6:
G-Spot Stimulation Techniques

Embarking on the journey of G-Spot stimulation can be an exhilarating and deeply enriching experience for those seeking to explore this nuanced aspect of sexual pleasure. To stimulate the G-Spot effectively, consider blending a variety of manual techniques, such as targeted pressure and rhythmic motions, with the use of specially designed toys that can enhance sensitivity and deliver intense feelings of ecstasy. It's not just about the mechanics, though; the emotional ambiance and mutual connection play pivotal roles. Experimentation and open communication are essential; each person is unique, and discovering what brings you or your partner the most pleasure can reveal new dimensions of intimacy and strengthen your bond. Whether you're journeying solo or with a partner, approaching this exploration with curiosity and positivity can lead to transformative sexual experiences. Remember, the goal is not solely orgasm but the journey of pleasure and connection.

manual techniques for the g-spot

Exploring G-Spot stimulation using manual techniques can open up a world of profound pleasure. It allows for intimate connection and communication between partners, or a deeper understanding of one's own body in solo play. The allure of manual stimulation lies in its versatility and the ability to finely tune one's touch, pressure, and rhythm based on immediate feedback. Whether you're looking to enhance your intimate relationship or explore solo, manual techniques serve as a foundation for discovering the G-Spot's full potential.

When it comes to locating the G-Spot, patience and exploration are key. The most common method involves having the receiving partner lie on their back with knees bent or legs spread apart. The giving partner can then insert one or two lubricated fingers into the vagina, curling them upward towards the navel to find a slightly rougher, ridged area on the front vaginal wall. This area, often identified as the G-Spot, may feel different from the surrounding tissue.

Another approach is to experiment with different positions. Having the receiving partner in a kneeling position, with the upper body lowered onto the bed, can provide a different angle for accessing the G-Spot. This variation can sometimes make it easier for both partners to engage in this intimate experience without straining or discomfort. Communication throughout the process is vital as it enhances the experience by adjusting movements and pressure to what's most pleasurable.

Once located, the G-Spot can be stimulated using direct pressure or rhythmic movements. Start gently, using a "come hither" motion with the fingers, applying steady pressure. Over time, gradually increase the intensity and speed according to the feedback from your partner. The G-Spot's sensitivity may vary, and this nuanced approach ensures comfort and pleasure are prioritized.

Manual techniques also benefit greatly from using lubricants. Enhanced lubrication reduces friction and increases comfort, allowing for more extended and enjoyable sessions. Water-based lubricants are often recommended as they are compatible with silicone toys and condoms if these are later incorporated into the session. Always keep a generous amount of lubricant on hand to maintain smooth and pleasurable movements.

Furthermore, incorporating other forms of touch and stimulation can amplify the overall experience. Light caresses on the inner thighs, clitoral stimulation, or gentle massaging of other erogenous zones can heighten arousal and intensify G-Spot sensations. This holistic approach treats the body as an interconnected system of pleasure points, enriching the experience and deepening the emotional connection between partners.

Communication remains a cornerstone of effective G-Spot stimulation. Open dialogs regarding preferences, boundaries, and sensations ensure that both partners feel comfortable and connected throughout the experience. Using verbal feedback and non-verbal cues like moans or changes in breath can help guide the stimulation towards what feels most pleasurable and satisfying.

Notably, the G-Spot can elicit a wide range of reactions. These can range from intense pleasure to emotional release. Some may experience a deep, fulfilling orgasm, while others might feel a buildup of pressure or even the urge to urinate due to the proximity to the bladder. Recognizing and validating these responses as natural parts of the journey helps normalize the experience and encourages a pressure-free exploration of pleasure.

If you're exploring solo, the same techniques apply. Use one or two fingers, employ a "come hither" motion, and vary the pressure and rhythm according to what feels best for you. Practicing alone can build a strong foundation of self-knowledge, which can be shared with a partner later. This self-awareness fosters confidence and eases the communication necessary for partnered play.

Some individuals enjoy alternating between steady pressure and rhythmic tapping on the G-Spot. Each technique offers its unique sensation - steady pressure might evoke a slow build-up of pleasure, while rhythmic tapping can provide quick bursts of intense sensation.

Mixing these techniques during a session keeps the experience dynamic and responsive to evolving arousal levels.

Incorporating Kegel exercises during G-Spot stimulation can further enhance the sensations. Kegels, which involve the contraction and relaxation of pelvic floor muscles, can increase internal pressure around the G-Spot and amplify pleasure. Regular practice of Kegel exercises not only boosts sexual pleasure but also promotes long-term pelvic health.

While manual techniques for G-Spot stimulation can stand alone as a powerful method, they also integrate beautifully with other forms of sexual activity. For example, combining G-Spot play with oral stimulation or intercourse can create layered sensations that lead to deeply satisfying blended orgasms. Adjusting positions during intercourse to align with G-Spot stimulation, like the modified missionary or cowgirl position, can seamlessly blend manual and penetrative pleasures.

Finally, it's important to approach G-Spot exploration with an attitude of curiosity and patience. Every individual's response to G-Spot stimulation is unique, and what works for one person might not work for another. Embrace the journey of discovering what feels right for you or your partner without the pressure to achieve a specific outcome. This openness enrichens the experience and fosters an environment of loving, exploratory connection.

Using Toys for G-Spot Pleasure

The realm of G-spot pleasure can be expanded significantly with the use of specially designed toys. While manual techniques provide an intimate, personal touch, the right toy can heighten sensations and offer sustained stimulation that might be challenging to achieve otherwise. Various toys have evolved to cater specifically to the intricate needs of G-spot pleasure, each bringing unique benefits and experiences to the table.

First and foremost, G-spot toys are typically designed with a specific curvature that allows for direct and precise stimulation of the G-spot. Located on the anterior wall of the vagina, approximately two to three inches inside, the G-spot responds well to firm, repetitive pressure. Toys designed for G-spot pleasure often have a pronounced curve or bulge at the end, aligning seamlessly with the body's natural contours to target this erogenous zone effectively.

When selecting a G-spot toy, material is a crucial consideration. Silicone is often recommended due to its body-safe properties, durability, and smooth texture. It's important to ensure that any toy used for G-spot stimulation is made from medical-grade silicone or other non-porous materials like glass or stainless steel. These materials are not only safe but also offer varied sensory experiences—glass and steel, for instance, can be warmed or cooled to add another layer of sensation.

Vibration is another feature common in G-spot toys that can elevate the experience dramatically. Vibrating G-spot toys come in many shapes and sizes, from slimline designs to more robust models. The vibrations can range from gentle pulses to intense throbs, providing diverse sensations that can help in exploring what feels best. Some G-spot vibrators also offer patterns, combining varying rhythms and intensities to keep the experience fresh and exciting.

In addition to vibrators, there are toys specifically called G-spot massagers. These tools are often ergonomically designed with a gentle curve and a broader head, which helps to distribute pressure more evenly across the G-spot. The sensation provided by a G-spot massager can feel more thorough and encompassing, often resulting in deeper and more prolonged pleasure.

Another popular option for G-spot stimulation is the use of dildos designed with a G-spot curve. These toys might not have vibration features but can offer substantial pleasure through manual control. Some individuals find that the self-paced, manual thrusting with a G-spot-curved dildo allows for more personalized control over their pleasure, making it possible to adjust pressure and speed according to preference.

For those interested in a dual-stimulation experience, there are rabbit vibrators and other dual-stim toys that provide both clitoral and G-spot stimulation simultaneously. These toys are particularly appreciated for their ability to blend different types of stimulation, potentially leading to blended orgasms—a combination of clitoral and G-spot orgasms—which can be immensely satisfying.

It's important to approach the use of G-spot toys with a sense of exploration and patience. Not every toy will work for every person, and preferences can vary widely. Experimenting with different shapes, sizes, and functions can be a delightful journey of discovering new facets of pleasure. Pay attention to how your body responds to different stimuli and make adjustments to find what feels most pleasurable.

Choosing the right setting and ambiance can enhance the experience with G-spot toys. Creating a relaxing environment with soft lighting, soothing music, and perhaps even aromatherapy can help set the mood and make the exploration process feel special and indulgent. Using a good quality water-based lubricant can also significantly enhance comfort and pleasure when using G-spot toys, making the experience smooth and enjoyable.

In addition to solo play, couples can also incorporate G-spot toys to enhance their shared intimacy. Introducing a G-spot toy during foreplay or intercourse can create new dimensions of pleasure and connection. Communicate openly with your partner about what feels good, and don't be afraid to guide them. The use of a toy can be a cooperative activity, deepening the bond between partners as they explore mutual pleasure.

In summary, G-spot toys offer an array of possibilities for enhancing sexual pleasure. Whether you're exploring solo or with a partner, the right toy can make an incredible difference in your intimate experiences. From vibrators to massagers to G-spot dildos, each tool has its unique attributes that cater to different needs and desires. Embrace the journey of exploration, and let these toys guide you to new heights of pleasure and satisfaction in your sexual life.

Chapter 7:
P-Spot Stimulation Techniques

Exploring P-Spot stimulation can open an incredible new realm of pleasure and intimacy for those willing to embark on this journey. To navigate this intimate terrain confidently, it's essential to understand both manual techniques and the use of toys specifically designed for this purpose. Start with gentle, exploratory touches using lubricated fingers, focusing on slow, rhythmic movements to build comfort and excitement. As you progress, toys tailored for P-Spot stimulation can enhance the experience, providing varied sensations that hands alone might not achieve. Communication, patience, and a willingness to experiment are key; these techniques can not only lead to powerful, satisfying orgasms but also deepen your connection with yourself or your partner. By embracing these methods, you'll empower yourself to unlock a dimension of sexual pleasure that is both deeply gratifying and transformative.

Manual Techniques for the P-Spot

Exploring manual techniques for P-Spot stimulation can open new vistas of pleasure and intimacy. Unlike other erogenous zones, the prostate or P-Spot has a unique set of considerations due to its anatomical position and sensitivity. Mastery of this involves understanding not just where the P-Spot is, but also how to approach it comfortably and effectively for both the giver and receiver.

The P-Spot is located approximately two to three inches inside the rectum, towards the front of the body. It feels slightly spongy and can be accessed by curving the finger in a 'come here' motion. For many men, this area can produce a new type of orgasm that is often described as deeply satisfying, intense, and prolonged.

Before diving into manual techniques, it's essential to create an environment of trust and open communication. Ensure both partners are comfortable with the concept and the process, discussing any boundaries and signals for continuing or stopping. This genuine connection can heighten the sense of safety and relaxation, allowing for a more enjoyable experience.

When preparing for P-Spot stimulation, hygiene is crucial. Cleanliness not only prevents infections but also helps put both partners at ease. Washing hands thoroughly and trimming fingernails can prevent accidental scratches. Using a lubricant is non-negotiable; the rectum doesn't produce its own lubrication, so a high-quality, water-based lubricant will make the experience more comfortable.

Begin with relaxation techniques to prepare the body. Deep breathing exercises and gentle massaging of surrounding areas, such as the buttocks and lower back, can help relax the muscles and enhance anticipation. For those new to this experience, starting with external stimulation around the anus can be beneficial. Light, circular motions can help the receiver identify and gradually become comfortable with the sensations.

Once both partners are relaxed and ready, the giver can slowly insert a well-lubricated finger, curving it slightly to reach the P-Spot. It's important to go slow, giving the receiver time to adjust to each new sensation. Gentle, consistent pressure can be applied to the P-Spot, with feedback from the receiver guiding the intensity and rhythm.

Some find that a rhythmic, massaging motion works best, while others may prefer gentle tapping or sustained pressure. It's essential to maintain open communication, discussing what feels good and what doesn't. Experimenting with different techniques can help discover the most pleasurable sensations for the receiver.

A common mistake is to focus solely on the prostate itself. Integrating whole-body touches can amplify the overall experience. For instance, combining prostate stimulation with simultaneous stimulation of the penis, nipples, or perineum can lead to powerful, blended orgasms. This holistic approach ensures that the entire body is engaged in the experience, enhancing intimacy and connection.

Encouraging relaxation and patience is key, particularly when new to P-Spot play. Rushing the process can lead to discomfort or even pain, which can create a negative association with what should be a pleasurable experience. Taking the time to explore and adjust to each sensation can lead to more profound enjoyment and connection.

Post-pleasure conversation is just as important as the act itself. Discussing what felt good, what could be improved, and any emotional responses can deepen the intimacy and trust between partners. This communication reinforces the connection and helps refine techniques for future encounters, paving the way for a fulfilling sexual journey together.

As you explore these manual techniques, be open to the evolving dynamics within your intimate relationship. Every individual's body responds differently, and preferences can change over time. By prioritizing mutual pleasure, communication, and trust, you create a shared space where both partners can feel empowered to experience the heights of P-Spot pleasure.

Ultimately, the journey of P-Spot exploration is about more than just physical pleasure. It's about deepening your bond, understanding each other's desires, and forging a path toward mutual satisfaction. By mastering these manual techniques, you're not only enriching your intimate life but also fostering a more profound emotional and physical connection.

Using Toys for P-Spot Pleasure

Incorporating toys into P-spot (prostate) stimulation can elevate the experience to unprecedented levels of pleasure. Prostate toys offer targeted sensation that manual techniques alone might be unable to achieve, opening doors to deeper, more consistent stimulation.

Prostate massagers are specifically designed with the male anatomy in mind. Their shapes are often curved to reach the P-spot effectively, with textures and vibrations that enhance the experience. Unlike general anal toys, prostate massagers are constructed to stimulate the prostate and are easy to use, even for beginners. They come in a variety of sizes and styles, catering to different experience levels and personal preferences. Some massagers have perineum stimulators, which provide additional external pleasure.

For those new to this type of stimulation, starting with a smaller, non-vibrating toy can make the process more comfortable and less intimidating. An initial focus on relaxation is crucial. Engage in a warm shower or bath beforehand to relax the muscles. Toys that are too large or intimidating can be discouraging, so choosing one that feels manageable is key. It's about finding a toy that feels right for your body and comfort level.

When it comes to lube, don't skimp. A generous application of water-based or silicone-based lubricant can make all the difference in comfort and ease of use. Since the anus does not lubricate itself naturally, lubrication is vital to prevent discomfort and potential injury. Some lubricants contain numbing agents, but caution is advised; one should always be able to listen to their body's signals.

The positioning of your body when using prostate toys matters too. Lying on your back with your knees bent, or on your side with one leg drawn up, can offer better access and comfort. Experiment with different positions to find what best suits your body's needs and preferences. Communication is essential, especially if you're not going solo. Expressing preferences and comfort levels with a partner can only enhance the experience.

Vibrating prostate massagers add another layer of pleasure that many find highly satisfying. These massagers come with different settings, from gentle pulsations to more vigorous vibrations. Experimenting with these settings can lead to a personalized and deeply enjoyable experience. Some toys even have remote controls, allowing for playful interaction between partners or easier adjustment if solo.

Rechargeable toys are another convenient feature to consider. They often offer stronger and more consistent vibrations compared to battery-operated options. Additionally, they tend to be more environmentally friendly, reducing the need for disposable batteries and ensuring the toy is always ready when you are.

Couples might find dual-stimulation toys particularly enjoyable, as they stimulate the prostate internally while providing external stimulation for the partner. These toys can make mutual play more engaging and satisfying, enhancing intimacy and connection. Coordinating the use of the toy with other forms of stimulation, like oral sex or manual techniques, can lead to explosive, blended orgasms.

When exploring prostate toys, cleanliness is non-negotiable. Toys should be cleaned before and after each use with antibacterial soap and water or a toy cleaner specifically designed for this purpose. Silicone toys should be stored in a clean, dry place to avoid any bacterial growth. It's also advisable to use condoms with shared toys to maintain hygiene and safety.

Once comfortable with the basics, one can explore more advanced toys and techniques. Rotating massagers provide a sweeping sensation across the prostate, potentially enhancing pleasure even further. Some advanced toys also offer heating capabilities, providing a soothing warmth that can enhance relaxation and arousal.

For some, the journey into prostate toy play might also include harnessing the mental aspects of pleasure. Visualization, breathing techniques, and being mentally present can take the physical sensations to an entirely new level. Combining these mental practices with the physical stimulation of a prostate massager can create an overwhelming and deeply satisfying experience.

Those who enjoy prostate play often speak of the powerful orgasms that can be achieved. These orgasms are often described as more intense and longer-lasting compared to penile-focused orgasms. The sensation originates deeper within the body, offering a full-bodied pleasure that engulfs the entire being. For many men, discovering this new realm of pleasure can be a transformative experience, altering their perspective on their own sexuality and intimacy.

Finally, remember that every individual's journey is unique. What works wonders for one person might not be as effective for another. The key is to remain open, curious, and willing to explore without judgment or high expectations. Prostate toy play is about discovering what brings the most pleasure and satisfaction to you and your partner.

The integration of toys into P-spot stimulation can be a thrilling and deeply enriching addition to one's sexual repertoire. By approaching this adventure with knowledge, patience, and a focus on shared or solo pleasure, the possibilities become boundless. Whether as a solo endeavour or as a shared intimate experience, the use of toys can offer unparalleled pleasure and connection, enhancing both physical sensations and emotional bonds.

Chapter 8:
Psychological Aspects of
G-Spot Stimulation

Exploring the psychological dimensions of G-Spot stimulation is as crucial as understanding the physical techniques, for the mind and body are intimately connected in the landscape of sexual pleasure. Embracing the power of one's mental state can create a harmonious experience where emotional readiness and physical sensations blend seamlessly. To fully enjoy G-Spot stimulation, it's essential to address and overcome any mental barriers that could hinder the experience, such as stress, shame, or insecurities. By nurturing a safe and open mindset, individuals and couples alike can amplify their pleasure and bond on a deeper level. Creating an environment of trust and communication enables a more fulfilling journey, where each touch and sensation is enhanced by the confidence and connection shared between partners. This holistic approach ensures that the mind is as prepared and eager as the body, fostering an enriching and unforgettable intimate adventure.

The Mind-Body Connection

When exploring the realm of sexual pleasure, one cannot overlook the profound link between the mind and body. Particularly in the context of G-Spot stimulation, the synchronization of mental and physical states plays a vital role in experiencing heightened pleasure and deeper intimacy. The mind-body connection is fundamental in transforming mere physical stimulation into a comprehensive, multi-dimensional experience.

The journey towards enriching one's sexual experiences begins in the mind. Mental states such as relaxation, focus, and openness significantly affect how the body responds to stimulation. For many, G-Spot stimulation is an unexplored territory, often shrouded in curiosity and even anxiety. Addressing these psychological components is crucial in unlocking its full potential. Intriguingly, the brain's involvement doesn't just stop at arousal; it encompasses the entire spectrum of sensations, emotions, and memories, crafting a fuller, richer narrative around each intimate encounter.

Mindfulness can be a powerful tool here. Engaging in mindfulness practices allows individuals to stay present, attuned to their bodies' sensations without judgment. Techniques such as deep breathing, visualization, and positive affirmations can act as gateways to relaxation, making it easier to reach the heightened states required for G-Spot pleasure. Imagine a scenario where the mind and body are harmoniously aligned—every stroke, every touch becomes exponentially more meaningful and pleasurable.

Often, the barriers to experiencing intense G-Spot pleasure lie within. Stress, past traumas, and societal pressures can create mental roadblocks. These influences can manifest as physical tension, making it difficult to relax and fully engage. Overcoming these barriers necessitates a compassionate and holistic approach. Cognitive-behavioral techniques, therapy, and even journaling about one's experiences and feelings related to sexuality can help dismantle these psychological obstacles.

The role of confidence can't be overstated. Feeling confident in one's body and sexuality can enhance the physiological arousal process. When individuals are confident, their bodies are likely more responsive, flexible, and receptive to new sensations. This self-assurance grows through education and self-exploration. Armed with knowledge about G-Spot stimulation and a willingness to experiment, individuals can foster a positive feedback loop: increased pleasure reinforces confidence, which in turn enhances physical responsiveness.

For couples, the mind-body connection bridges not only individual experiences but shared ones as well. Open, honest communication about desires, boundaries, and fantasies deepens emotional intimacy, which translates into more gratifying physical intimacy. Discussing likes, dislikes, and curiosities in a safe, non-judgmental space can significantly elevate the quality of sexual interaction. Mutual exploration fosters trust, allowing both partners to feel secure enough to lose themselves in the experience.

For some, cultural and societal conditioning may have shaped their views about sexuality in restrictive ways. Unlearning these barriers involves both awareness and active effort. It might be helpful to engage with resources that normalize and celebrate sexual exploration, thereby fostering a more liberating mindset.

Visualization is another potent technique. This involves mentally rehearsing the pleasurable scenarios one wishes to experience. Visualization can prime the brain to recognize and amplify the sensations associated with G-Spot stimulation, effectively creating a blueprint for pleasure. Such practices allow individuals to bridge the gap between fantasy and reality, making what once seemed unattainable entirely possible.

The concept of neuroplasticity supports the potent relationship between the mind and body. The brain's ability to reorganize itself by forming new neural connections means that cultivating positive sexual experiences can lead to sustained improvements in sexual health and pleasure. Through continual practice and positive reinforcement, individuals can train their brains to associate G-Spot stimulation with profound pleasure.

This intimate mind-body synergy encourages a holistic approach to sexual health, acknowledging that pleasure and wellness are not just facets of physical existence but are deeply rooted in our mental well-being. To truly harness the pleasure potential of the G-Spot, one must cultivate mental resilience, emotional openness, and a compassionate understanding of their own needs and desires.

Thus, the pursuit of G-Spot stimulation isn't just about discovering a pleasure point but about fostering a deeper connection with oneself. It's a journey of understanding how the mind can elevate physical sensations to create a more profound, enriching sexual experience. By recognizing and nurturing this mind-body connection, individuals and couples can embark on a holistic path to sexual wellness, filled with discovery, intimacy, and abundant pleasure.

Overcoming Mental Barriers

Exploring new facets of sexual pleasure, especially something as specific as G-Spot stimulation, requires not just physical readiness but also a significant mental and emotional preparedness. The very idea might evoke a variety of emotions, from excitement to anxiety. To truly engage in this form of intimate exploration, it is crucial to address and overcome any mental barriers that may hinder the experience.

Mental barriers often stem from societal conditioning, past experiences, or personal insecurities. Many people grow up with rigid ideas about sexuality, leading to hesitancy and discomfort with trying new things. It's important to recognize that these barriers are entirely normal but shouldn't dictate your sexual discovery. Understanding and addressing them can pave the way for a more fulfilling intimate life.

One common mental barrier is the fear of inadequacy. The belief that you might not "do it right" can be paralyzing. It's important to remember that sexual exploration, including G-Spot stimulation, is a journey rather than a destination. There is no perfect way to explore your body or your partner's. The key lies in communication and a willingness to learn together. Embrace the imperfections; they're part of what makes the experience unique and personal.

Shame and guilt, often rooted in cultural or religious backgrounds, can also be significant obstacles. These feelings can create a mental block that dampens sexual curiosity. Overcoming this requires a shift in perspective; seeing sexual pleasure as a natural, healthy part of human experience rather than something to be hidden or suppressed. Reading and learning about the anatomy and function of the G-Spot can help demystify it and reduce feelings of shame.

Another mental barrier might be the fear of pain or discomfort. You've perhaps read or been told that G-Spot stimulation can be intense and might even be uncomfortable until you become accustomed to it. This is a valid concern, but addressing it involves both physical technique and mental readiness. Start gently and listen to your body, allowing yourself to acclimate gradually. Turn your focus inward; meditate on the sensations and allow your body to guide you. Visualization techniques can also greatly aid in easing into this new experience.

Self-consciousness about body image or performance can diminish the joy of exploring G-Spot stimulation. Many people get tangled in thoughts about how they look or how they're performing, which can detract from the overall experience. Practicing self-compassion and engaging in positive self-talk can help shift your focus from how you appear to what you feel. Remind yourself that the beauty of this journey lies in the pleasure and connection, not in meeting some external standard of attractiveness or performance.

Anxiety can be another formidable barrier. The anticipation of trying something new, particularly something as intimate as G-Spot exploration, can generate considerable stress. Learning relaxation techniques such as deep breathing, mindfulness, or engaging in a soothing pre-intimacy ritual can alleviate anxiety. Setting a serene, comfortable environment free from distractions will also help create a sense of calm and readiness.

One often-overlooked mental barrier is the "busyness" of modern life. A crowded mind, preoccupied with daily stresses and responsibilities, can find it challenging to get into the right headspace for intimate exploration. Allocating intentional time for sexual and emotional connection with yourself or your partner can help mitigate this barrier. Make space in your schedule, no matter how busy; consider this time as a necessary investment in your well-being.

Communication plays a pivotal role in overcoming mental barriers, especially in partnered scenarios. Discussing your fears, concerns, and desires with your partner can alleviate much of the anxiety associated with G-Spot exploration. It also fosters mutual understanding and empathy, strengthening the emotional connection between you. The same principle applies to solo exploration; communicating openly with yourself through journaling or self-reflection can help identify and dismantle these barriers.

For those who find it exceptionally challenging to overcome mental barriers, professional help can be an invaluable resource. Therapists who specialize in sexual health and therapy can provide personalized strategies and a supportive space to work through these issues. Don't hesitate to seek out this form of guidance if you feel it might benefit you.

In some cases, mental barriers are linked to past traumas or negative sexual experiences. Whether it's a result of abuse, coercion, or an emotionally painful encounter, these experiences leave deep psychological imprints. Overcoming such barriers requires immense care and often professional support. Trauma-informed therapy can offer the necessary tools and techniques to heal and reclaim your sense of sexual agency.

So, how can you mentally prepare yourself for exploring G-Spot stimulation? Consider starting with education. Knowledge truly is power. Understanding the anatomy, the science behind G-Spot stimulation, and reading about others' experiences can demystify the process. There's something incredibly empowering about knowing what to expect and having a clear understanding of the sensations involved.

Visualization exercises can also be helpful. Before you engage in physical exploration, take time to visualize a positive and pleasurable experience. Close your eyes, breathe deeply, and imagine the sensations, the pleasure, the warmth, and the connection. This mental rehearsal can set a hopeful and positive tone for the actual encounter.

Finally, adopt a mindset of curiosity and playfulness. Sexual exploration, especially something as specific as G-Spot stimulation, should be seen as a delightful adventure rather than a task to be perfected. Curiosity liberates you from the tyranny of expectations. Playfulness allows joy to take center stage, creating an experience that's both fun and fulfilling. Remember, the journey is uniquely yours, and every discovery along the way enriches your understanding and intimacy.

Embracing a holistic approach, acknowledging your mental barriers, and methodically addressing them can transform your exploration of G-Spot stimulation into a truly enlightening experience. It's about creating a space where you feel safe, accepted, and free to experience pleasure. By overcoming these mental barriers, you're not just enhancing your sexual pleasure; you're also engaging in a profound act of self-love and empowerment.

Chapter 9:
Psychological Aspects of
P-Spot Stimulation

Understanding the psychological aspects of P-Spot stimulation is crucial for a fulfilling experience. The journey begins with emotional and mental preparedness, where embracing vulnerability and openness can transform apprehension into anticipation. In the realm of intimate exploration, building a context of trust and comfort paves the way for deeper connection and pleasure. Partner communication is essential; expressing desires and boundaries candidly fosters a shared space of mutual respect and emotional safety. This dialogue not only demystifies the experience but also enhances intimacy, allowing both partners to navigate the nuances of P-Spot pleasure with confidence and curiosity. When mind and body synchronize in this dance of exploration, the potential for profound satisfaction and connection is boundless.

Emotional and Mental Preparedness

Stepping into the realm of P-Spot stimulation can be a thrilling and enlightening journey. However, before diving into the physical techniques, it's essential to address the emotional and mental preparedness necessary for a fulfilling experience. Understanding this aspect sets a strong foundation, ensuring that exploration is not only enjoyable but also psychologically enlightening.

The first step is to cultivate a sense of curiosity and openness about the experience. Sexual pleasure, especially when involving lesser-known erogenous zones like the P-Spot, requires a mindset free from stigma and preconceived notions. This openness allows you to approach new sensations without fear or judgment, creating an environment where pleasure can flourish. Curiosity drives the exploration, but acceptance and open-mindedness foster lasting satisfaction and psychological well-being.

Many people carry societal and cultural baggage when it comes to anal play, and the P-Spot is no exception. It's crucial to confront any internalized shame or discomfort head-on. Societal norms and misinformation can often lead to negative feelings about P-Spot stimulation, branding it as taboo or inappropriate. Recognizing that these ideas are rooted in ignorance can be liberating. By shedding these irrational fears and embracing a more informed perspective, you set yourself up for more meaningful and pleasurable experiences.

An essential part of mental readiness involves understanding one's own body and its potential for pleasure. This might start with some solo exploration, giving you the chance to learn and appreciate your body's responses at your own pace. Doing so in a safe and private space can significantly reduce anxiety, allowing you to better grasp what feels good and what doesn't. This personal journey is empowering, equipping you with the knowledge and confidence required to further explore intimate connections with a partner.

In relationships, emotional preparedness extends to communication and trust with your partner. Open, honest dialogues about desires and boundaries are non-negotiable. Talking about expectations and concerns can eliminate misunderstandings and create a mutual sense of security. This foundation of trust allows both partners to engage in P-Spot stimulation without fear of judgement, creating a shared space where pleasure and intimacy can thrive.

Moreover, it's important to highlight that patience is a virtue in this journey. Emotional readiness doesn't happen overnight. For some, the idea of P-Spot stimulation might evoke a mix of excitement and apprehension. Taking the time to educate oneself, discussing with one's partner, and engaging in mindful practices can help ease into the experience. Meditation or mindfulness exercises can be beneficial in managing any underlying anxiety, allowing for a more relaxed and receptive state of mind.

Maintaining a compassionate attitude towards oneself is equally critical. It's entirely normal to feel a spectrum of emotions—from excitement to nervousness—about exploring the P-Spot. Self-compassion means acknowledging these feelings without judgment, understanding that emotional reactions are part of the human experience. When you accept your emotions, you create a supportive internal environment that encourages exploration without undue stress.

Therapy or counseling can also be helpful, particularly for those who have experienced trauma related to their sexuality or have deep-seated anxieties. A professional can provide strategies to navigate these emotions constructively, ensuring that past experiences don't hinder current and future pleasures. Understanding that mental health and sexual well-being are intertwined underscores the importance of addressing psychological factors in any sexual exploration.

Another vital aspect of emotional and mental preparedness is the practice of setting and respecting boundaries. This involves clearly defining what you are and are not comfortable with before engaging in P-Spot play. Boundaries protect your emotional and physical well-being, ensuring that any explorative activities are consensual and mutually enjoyable. Being upfront about your limits with yourself and your partner leads to more satisfying and secure experiences.

Visualization and affirmations are practical tools for mental readiness. Visualizing a successful and pleasurable experience can create a positive mindset, while affirmations reinforce self-assurance and confidence. Phrases like "I am capable of experiencing deep pleasure" or "I respect and honor my boundaries" can be powerful in reshaping the mental landscape towards positivity and readiness for new sexual experiences.

Additionally, creating a conducive environment for exploration can significantly impact your emotional state. A comfortable, private, and aesthetically pleasing space can enhance relaxation and openness. Soft lighting, soothing music, and comfortable bedding are minor adjustments that can have a substantial effect on your mindset, helping to create a sanctuary for pleasure and connection.

Emotional preparedness also involves reflecting on past sexual experiences and understanding how they shape your current feelings about P-Spot stimulation. Positive and negative past experiences both provide valuable insights. Reflecting on these can help identify what you may need more of, less of, or entirely different approaches for current and future explorations. This reflective practice encourages growth, ensuring that each new experience builds on a foundation of self-awareness and informed choices.

In conclusion, emotional and mental preparedness for P-Spot stimulation is a multifaceted process. It involves a mix of self-education, open-mindedness, trust-building, and self-compassion. By addressing and nurturing these aspects, you create a solid foundation for not just P-Spot pleasure, but a deeper, more empowering understanding of your sexual self and intimate connections.

Partner Communication

Communication is the cornerstone of any intimate relationship, more so when exploring something as personal and profound as P-spot stimulation. It's essential to approach these conversations with sensitivity and openness. Often, the most challenging aspect is initiating the dialogue. Expressing curiosity and willingness to explore new dimensions of pleasure can set a positive tone. Remember, it's not just about what you say but how you say it.

One effective approach is to frame the conversation around mutual exploration and learning. Phrases like "I've been reading about P-spot stimulation and I think it could be really enjoyable for both of us" can invite your partner into a collaborative journey. Emphasize that this is about enriching your shared experiences, not just fulfilling a personal curiosity. This way, the conversation feels inclusive rather than confrontational.

It's also important to listen. Be mindful of your partner's feelings and reactions. They might have reservations or questions, and addressing these openly can strengthen trust. For example, they might be concerned about hygiene or discomfort. Validate these concerns and provide information to address them—detail later chapters such as "Safety and Hygiene for P-Spot Stimulation" can be particularly helpful here. In this dialogue, patience is key.

Creating a safe space for these conversations often means choosing the right time and setting. A relaxed environment where you're not pressed for time can significantly impact how the discussion unfolds. Expressing your thoughts during a quiet evening at home, rather than in a rushed or public setting, can lead to more meaningful exchanges. Physical intimacy, like cuddling or holding hands, can also be a great backdrop for these talks—it helps in building a sense of closeness and safety.

Non-verbal communication should not be underestimated either. Our bodies often speak volumes. Maintaining eye contact, offering reassuring touches, and displaying relaxed body language can make a world of difference. These non-verbal cues reinforce the idea that this exploration is a shared and desired experience. In this sense, actions truly do complement words.

Another aspect to consider is the use of positive reinforcement. When your partner expresses any willingness to discuss or try P-spot stimulation, acknowledge their openness and thank them for considering it. Positive feedback can foster a protective and loving space where both partners feel valued and respected.

It's also beneficial to share educational resources. Sending an article, a book recommendation, or even watching a documentary together can provide a shared learning experience. This also shows that you're both committed to understanding and enhancing your intimate relationship. Sometimes, having a third-party source explain the benefits and mechanics of P-spot stimulation can make the subject easier to approach.

Setting boundaries is critical. Consent is at the heart of any sexual exploration, and P-spot stimulation is no exception. Discussing what each partner is comfortable with before diving in can prevent misunderstandings and ensure a pleasurable experience for both. It's prudent to establish a safe word or signals that will immediately stop any activity if one partner feels uncomfortable. This creates a foundation of trust and reassurance.

It's also important to revisit and reevaluate your conversations regularly. People's comfort levels and desires can change over time; what felt acceptable or intriguing at one point might need to be renegotiated later. Keeping the dialogue open ensures that both partners remain on the same page and can adapt as necessary.

In developing this habit of open communication, partners often find that their relationship deepens not just sexually but emotionally. Discussing intimate desires and boundaries fosters a sense of vulnerability and trust that enriches the overall connection. This practice of mutual respect and understanding transcends the bedroom, benefiting various facets of the relationship.

In situations where one partner finds it particularly challenging to discuss, couples' therapy can also be a valuable resource. A professional can help navigate these conversations, providing tools and frameworks that make the dialogue more manageable. Sometimes an external perspective can bridge gaps that seem otherwise insurmountable.

Ultimately, effective partner communication about P-spot stimulation builds a stronger, more connected intimate relationship. It's about exploration, understanding, and mutual respect. As you and your partner embark on this journey, remember that the path is as meaningful as the destination. It's in these moments of connection and communication that true intimacy and pleasure are found.

In conclusion, thoughtful and open communication paves the way for a more profound and rewarding sexual relationship. Embrace these conversations, approach them with sensitivity, and remain open to where they might lead. It's through this process that you will discover new dimensions of pleasure and connection, enriching your relationship in truly transformative ways.

Chapter 10:
G-Spot Stimulation for Solo Play

The exploration of G-spot stimulation during solo play can be an incredibly empowering and exhilarating journey. It requires a blend of curiosity, patience, and self-awareness, inviting you to tune into your body's unique rhythms and sensations. Start by finding a comfortable and private setting where you can fully immerse yourself in this intimate discovery. Use your fingers or a specially designed toy, experimenting with gentle pressure and rhythmic movements as you explore different angles and techniques. As you focus on your internal sensations, remember that the journey itself is just as significant as the destination. Listen to your body's responses and let your pleasure guide you, trusting that with each moment of mindful exploration, you are uncovering new and profound layers of your sexual self-awareness. Isn't it breathtaking to realize the vast potential of pleasure that lies within your own fingertips?

Enhancing Personal Pleasure

The journey of exploring personal pleasure through G-spot stimulation is as thrilling as it is enlightening. While the G-spot, or Gräfenberg spot, has long been the subject of fascination and debate, its potential to unlock profound pleasure is undeniable. Venturing into G-spot stimulation for solo play can be a transformative experience, allowing you to deepen your self-awareness and tap into new realms of sensual delight.

One of the first steps in enhancing personal pleasure is creating a comfortable and safe environment where you can explore without distractions. Your physical surroundings play an important role in setting the tone. Dim lighting, soft music, and perhaps a scented candle can turn your space into a sanctuary of self-love. The goal is to make yourself feel at ease, creating a mental and physical landscape that invites relaxation and exploration.

Breathing deeply and allowing your mind to settle is essential. Engaging in mindful practices can greatly enhance your sensitivity and responsiveness. Take a moment to breathe, feeling each inhalation deeply and letting go of tension with every exhalation. When you're present in your body, your mind becomes more attuned to subtle sensations, which can elevate your entire experience.

When it comes to the techniques themselves, understanding and experimenting are key. Begin with gentle exploration. Using your fingers, apply light pressure, and notice the varying textures and sensations. Listen to your body, paying close attention to which movements and pressures elicit the most pleasure. Finding a rhythm that resonates with you can make a world of difference.

Variation in techniques is crucial. Don't be afraid to experiment with pace and intensity. Some might find a slow, rhythmic motion more pleasurable, while others might prefer a faster, more persistent stimulation. Trust your intuition and explore different approaches to see what feels best for you.

Using toys can significantly enhance personal pleasure. Designed specifically to target the G-spot, these toys can offer more precision and consistency. Whether you choose a curved vibrator or a G-spot wand, explore different devices and their settings. Make sure to use plenty of lubrication to heighten sensations and reduce any discomfort. Remember, there's no rush; take your time to discover what works best for you.

Incorporating clitoral stimulation might amplify G-spot pleasure, leading to blended orgasms that many describe as mind-blowing. Combining internal and external stimulation can create a feedback loop of pleasure, where each type of stimulation enhances the other. There are dual-stimulation toys available, but you can also use a separate vibrator or your fingers for clitoral pleasure.

Taking time to explore your bodily responses is a powerful way to enhance personal pleasure. Notice how your body reacts to different touches, and don't hesitate to change methods if something doesn't feel right. Your body's feedback is the most valuable guide in this journey. Enjoy the exploration process, savoring the sensations without focusing solely on the end goal of orgasm. Sometimes, the journey itself can be just as satisfying.

Consider incorporating different positions to see how they impact your pleasure. Lying on your back with your knees bent, or squatting, can change the angle and pressure on the G-spot. Positions that allow your body to fully relax, yet provide easy access, can make the experience more comfortable and pleasurable.

As you delve deeper into this intimate practice, maintaining an open mind and embracing curiosity can reveal unexpected pleasures. Personal pleasure is highly individual, shaped by your unique anatomy and preferences. Embrace the trial-and-error nature of this exploration, and don't be discouraged by initial difficulties. The more you practice, the more in tune you'll become with your body's signals.

Emotional readiness and self-compassion are just as important as physical techniques. Approaching this journey with a loving and compassionate attitude towards oneself can create a nurturing space where true pleasure thrives. Remember, this is about your enjoyment and empowerment. Celebrate each discovery and be gentle with yourself during times of frustration or sensitivity.

It's also beneficial to educate oneself about the scientific basis of G-spot stimulation. Knowledge about the structures and functions involved can dispel myths and misconceptions, making your exploration more informed and effective. Understanding how the G-spot connects to other erogenous zones can provide a more comprehensive approach to solo play.

In summary, enhancing personal pleasure through G-spot stimulation is a multifaceted journey that involves creating a conducive environment, experimenting with different techniques and toys, incorporating mindfulness practices, and maintaining an open, curious attitude. This intimate exploration not only deepens your self-awareness but also empowers you to experience new heights of pleasure. Celebrate this personal journey, knowing that each step brings you closer to understanding the depths of your sensual potential.

Exploring Different Techniques

When it comes to solo exploration of G-Spot stimulation, the key lies in discovering what feels best for your unique body. Every individual will have different preferences, and the journey is all about finding what brings you the most pleasure. As we embark on this exploration, it's essential to remain patient, curious, and open to experimenting with various techniques. Remember, this is a personal voyage of self-discovery.

First and foremost, preparing your mind and body for this exploration is crucial. Setting the mood can significantly enhance your experience. Dim the lights, play some relaxing music, and ensure that you're in a comfortable and private space where you won't be disturbed. Allowing your mind to relax and your body to follow will create a more conducive environment for your journey. This step shouldn't be overlooked, as it establishes the foundation for a more fulfilling experience.

One of the most effective techniques to explore is the use of your fingers. Start by gently caressing the external parts of your vulva to increase arousal and ensure your vaginal canal is sufficiently lubricated. As you become more aroused, insert a well-lubricated finger (or fingers) into the vagina, curling it in a 'come-hither' motion towards the front wall of the vaginal canal. The G-Spot is typically located about two to three inches inside. Gentle, rhythmic motions or light pressure can start the stimulation process.

Feeling the texture of the G-Spot, which can often be described as slightly ridged or spongy, can guide you in understanding how your body responds. Some people may prefer a consistent, steady pressure, while others might enjoy a more varied rhythm, alternating between tapping, massaging, and swirling motions. Pay attention to how your body reacts and trust your intuition to adjust the technique accordingly.

Alongside manual techniques, incorporating sex toys designed specifically for G-Spot stimulation can be incredibly beneficial. Toys like G-Spot vibrators or curved dildos are crafted to reach and massage the G-Spot effectively. These toys provide a range of vibration patterns and intensities, allowing you to experiment and find what feels best. An advantage of using toys is that they can maintain consistent pressure and offer varied sensations that might be harder to achieve manually.

When using toys, apply a generous amount of lubricant to both the toy and your vaginal opening. This will ensure a smooth, pleasurable experience and reduce the risk of discomfort or irritation. Begin with slower, gentler movements, gradually increasing intensity as you become more aroused and comfortable. The goal is to find a rhythm that resonates with your body's responses.

Breathwork is another often overlooked yet highly effective technique to enhance G-Spot stimulation. Deep, intentional breathing can help you stay present and connected to your body, intensifying the sensations. As you stimulate the G-Spot, synchronize your breath with your movements. Inhale deeply as you press or massage, and exhale slowly to relax and release any tension. This synchronicity amplifies the connection between your mind and body, elevating the overall experience.

Exploring different positions can also significantly affect the sensations you experience. While lying on your back with your knees bent and legs apart is a common starting point, don't hesitate to experiment with positions like squatting, standing with one leg elevated, or even lying on your stomach. Each position offers a different angle and depth of penetration, potentially unlocking new levels of pleasure.

Incorporating pelvic floor exercises, such as Kegels, into your routine can also enhance G-Spot stimulation. Strong pelvic floor muscles can provide greater control and intensity during stimulation, leading to more satisfying orgasms. Regularly practicing these exercises will increase your ability to contract and relax these muscles, giving you better control over your body's responses during G-Spot play.

Visual or mental stimulation can further heighten the physical sensations you experience. Engaging your mind with erotic fantasies, reading erotica, or watching consensual adult content can enhance arousal and intensify your experience. Embracing your sexual fantasies without judgment and allowing them to play a role in your solo exploration can be incredibly empowering and liberating.

Don't underestimate the power of combining G-Spot stimulation with other forms of arousal. Blending G-Spot play with clitoral stimulation, either manually or with a dual-action toy, can lead to incredibly intense and fulfilling orgasms. Clitoral stimulation can heighten overall arousal, making the G-Spot more sensitive and responsive. The combined sensations create a symphony of pleasure, sometimes culminating in what is known as a blended orgasm, which taps into multiple erogenous zones simultaneously.

It's also crucial to be mindful of how your body communicates its needs and limits. If certain techniques cause discomfort, it's okay to stop and try something else. The goal is to enjoy the experience, not to force it. Listen to your body, adjust as needed, and remember that sometimes the journey might be more about exploration and less about reaching a specific destination.

Lastly, maintaining a positive and non-judgmental attitude towards your exploration can make all the difference. Everyone's journey is unique, and what works for one person might not work for another. Celebrate your progress, however small it may seem, and recognize that sexual self-discovery is a continual process. Embrace the curiosity and delight in the moments of newfound pleasure and connection with your body.

As you continue to explore different techniques, remember that patience and self-compassion are your best allies. Give yourself permission to experiment without self-imposed pressure or expectations. Over time, you'll develop a deeper understanding of your body and its responses, paving the way for richer, more fulfilling solo sessions that celebrate your sexual autonomy and pleasure.

Chapter 11:
P-Spot Stimulation for Solo Play

Embarking on the journey of P-spot stimulation solo allows you to intimately discover your body's responses and pleasures, guided purely by your own pace and comfort. Delve into personal exploration with patience and curiosity; the prostate, often referred to as the P-spot, harbors potential for intense, mind-blowing orgasms. Start by familiarizing yourself with the area using well-lubricated fingers or a specially designed P-spot toy. Experiment with different angles and pressures, paying attention to how your body reacts. It may take time to initially find and stimulate the P-spot effectively, but each session is an opportunity to learn more about what brings you pleasure. Remember, relaxation is key—set a serene atmosphere, focus on your breathing, and let each sensation guide you to the next. The combination of physical touch and mental arousal can create a magnificent symphony of pleasure, giving you a deeper connection to your sexual wellbeing.

Personal Exploration

Embarking on a journey of personal exploration, especially when it comes to understanding your own sexual pleasure, can be both an enlightening and deeply gratifying experience. Solo play focusing on P-spot stimulation offers an opportunity not just for intimate satisfaction but also for a closer connection with your own desires and body. It's an invitation to understand the nuances of what generates pleasure and how your body responds to various forms of touch.

Firstly, it's essential to create an atmosphere where you feel both comfortable and safe. Privacy is key, as you want to fully immerse yourself in the moment without any interruptions. Consider setting the scene with soft lighting, maybe some soothing music, and elements that make the environment feel inviting and calm. This mindfulness in preparation can make a significant difference in how receptive your body will be.

Before diving into the mechanics of P-spot stimulation, it's vital to connect with your body on a fundamental level. Taking time to explore your body without any specific goal in mind can be incredibly revealing. Use your hands to trace along your skin, allowing yourself to experience different textures and pressures. This process is not just a warm-up; it's also a form of training, helping you build awareness of how your body reacts to different stimuli.

Breathing exercises can further enhance your personal exploration. Deep, rhythmic breathing helps in relaxing your body and mind. As you take in each breath, imagine that you're drawing in positive energy, filling yourself with calm and focus. Exhaling, let go of any tension or distractions that might be lingering. This practice facilitates a state of mindfulness, making you more attuned to the sensations you're about to experience.

As you prepare for P-spot stimulation, lubrication is an absolute necessity. The tissues involved are delicate, and ample lubrication ensures that your exploration is both comfortable and pleasurable. Choose a high-quality lubricant that is compatible with your needs, whether it's water-based, silicone-based, or another suitable option.

Starting with external stimulation can be a gentle segue into your exploration. Use your fingers to massage the perineum, the area located between the testicles and the anus. This region is sensitive and can be a highly pleasurable zone in its own right. Experiment with varying pressures and movements, listening to how your body responds. This form of external massage can serve as both an introduction and a teaser, building anticipation for deeper exploration.

When you're ready to move internally, consider your posture. Positions that offer you comfort and ease of access are ideal. Many find that lying on their back with knees bent, or squatting, provides the optimal angles for reaching the P-spot. Remember that there is no one-size-fits-all approach—experiment to find what feels right for you.

Gently insert a well-lubricated finger or a specifically designed toy. The P-spot, or prostate gland, is located about two inches inside the rectum, towards the front of the body. It's essential to move slowly and be mindful of your comfort level. There's no rush; exploration is about savoring the experience rather than racing towards a particular outcome.

Techniques for Stimulation:

Once you've identified the P-spot, experiment with different techniques to discover what brings you the most pleasure. Gentle tapping, circular motions, or steady pressure can elicit varying sensations. Some may find a come-hither motion particularly pleasurable. The key is to pay attention to your body's feedback, adjusting your movements accordingly.

As you grow more comfortable and familiar with P-spot stimulation, you can start integrating other forms of stimulation. Combining P-spot touch with penile stimulation, for example, can amplify sensations and lead to intense orgasms. The dual stimulation engages multiple pleasure centers simultaneously, creating a fuller and more immersive experience.

The psychological component of personal exploration is equally significant. Embrace an open-minded and non-judgmental attitude towards your body and its responses. Exploring your own sexual pleasure is as much about understanding your mental and emotional landscape as it is about physical sensations. This journey can uncover not just what brings you pleasure but also deeper insights into your own sexuality and desires.

Furthermore, taking notes or keeping a journal about your experiences can help you map out what techniques and practices work best for you. Document your journey, not just the physical details but also your emotional and psychological responses. This reflective practice can provide valuable insights over time and help you to continuously refine and enhance your solo play.

Engaging in personal exploration doesn't end with a single successful session. It's an ongoing journey, with each experience adding layers to your understanding of your own body. Allow yourself to grow from each session, seeing it as part of a larger narrative of self-discovery and sexual empowerment. Experimentation and consistency will bring a deeper connection to your desires, leading to a more fulfilling and nuanced understanding of pleasure.

By fully immersing yourself in personal exploration with an open heart and mind, you enable the creation of a space where genuine, uninhibited pleasure can flourish. It's not just about reaching an orgasm; it's about the entire experience of feeling, understanding, and celebrating your body's capabilities.

So, delve into your personal exploration with curiosity and respect for yourself. The knowledge you gain from these intimate moments alone is invaluable, laying the foundation for richer and more profound sexual experiences, whether solo or partnered. Always remember, the journey of understanding your own pleasure is uniquely yours and endlessly rewarding.

Techniques for Maximum Pleasure

Achieving maximum pleasure from P-Spot stimulation can be a journey of discovery filled with both excitement and deep satisfaction.

For those new to this experience, it might feel intimidating, but remember, the key lies in confidence, patience, and a willingness to explore. Begin with an open mind and a relaxed body.

First, it's crucial to create a comfortable and tranquil environment. Ambient lighting, soft music, and a warm setting can set the mood, helping you relax physically and mentally. Comfort aids in diminishing any initial tension or apprehension you may have about exploring your P-Spot.

Start with basic relaxation techniques. Breathing exercises can significantly reduce anxiety. Take deep, measured breaths and allow your body to settle into a state of calm. This practice can also help you tune into your body's responses, making you more aware of subtle sensations as you begin your exploration.

Lubrication is non-negotiable when it comes to P-Spot stimulation. Use a generous amount of water-based or silicone-based lubricant to ensure smooth and comfortable movements. The anal area doesn't self-lubricate, so ample lubrication is essential for both comfort and safety.

When you feel ready, you can begin by gently massaging the perineum, the sensitive area between the scrotum and the anus. This can serve as a warm-up, enhancing blood flow and increasing arousal. It's a good introduction to the sensations that lie ahead.

Using your finger initially can give you greater control and a better feel for what you're comfortable with. Slowly and gently insert a lubricated finger into the anus with a "come-hither" motion directed towards the navel. With patience and a gentle approach, you'll feel the prostate, a walnut-sized gland located about 2 inches inside. It may feel like a firm, rounded bump.

Patience is key. Don't rush; take your time exploring the different textures and pressures that feel pleasurable. Some might feel an immediate surge of pleasure, while for others, it may take a bit more time and exploration to hit the right spot. It's a personal journey, and no two experiences are identical.

Introduce toys gradually. Prostate massagers, anal beads, or butt plugs specifically designed for P-Spot stimulation can enhance the experience once you're comfortable with manual exploration. Select products made from body-safe materials like medical-grade silicone. Begin with smaller sizes and gradually work up as you gain confidence and familiarity with the sensations.

Incorporate varied speeds and pressures. Change the rhythm of your touches and movements to discover what intensifies your pleasure. Some may prefer a steady, consistent pressure, while others might crave a more dynamic, pulsing sensation. Listen to your body and adjust accordingly.

Simultaneously stimulating other erogenous zones can amplify your experience. Combine P-Spot stimulation with manual penile stimulation or nipple play. These dual sensations can create a more intense and pleasurable experience, often leading to more powerful orgasms.

Experiment with different positions. Lying on your back with your knees bent and legs apart can offer easy access. Alternatively, some might find more comfort and control by squatting. Each position provides a unique angle and pressure on the P-Spot, so find what works best for your body.

Focus on relaxation and mindfulness. The more relaxed your body is, the easier it will be to enjoy P-Spot stimulation. Mindfulness can help you fully experience each sensation and stay in tune with what feels best.

It's essential to stay hydrated and be aware of your body's limits. Overstimulation can cause discomfort, so if at any point something feels off, don't hesitate to pause or stop. It's crucial to listen to and respect your body's signals.

Using a mirror can be helpful for understanding the process visually. It can confirm you're approaching the correct areas and applying suitable pressure. This visual aid can be particularly helpful for beginners who might be uncertain about their technique.

Journaling your experiences can be beneficial. Documenting what worked, what didn't, and how different techniques felt can provide insights for future sessions. Over time, you'll refine your technique and discover new paths to pleasure.

Building mental arousal alongside physical stimulation can deepen the overall experience. Fantasies, erotic literature, or visual stimuli can heighten your arousal and sync your mind with the sensations your body is experiencing.

Understand that reaching an orgasm through P-Spot stimulation might not happen immediately. This process can require practice and a deeper understanding of your body. Celebrate small victories and enjoy the journey without fixating on the endpoint.

Ultimately, the goal is self-discovery and the enhanced pleasure that comes with it. Respect your pace, and recognize that every step forward is a step towards greater intimacy with yourself. Mastering these techniques takes time, patience, and a spirit of exploration, but the journey is immensely gratifying.

Chapter 12:
G-Spot Stimulation for Couples

Exploring G-Spot stimulation as a couple can enhance intimacy and trust, turning physical pleasure into a shared journey of discovery. Through open communication and mutual understanding, partners can dive into this form of pleasure together, finding new layers of connection and excitement. Consider experimenting with different positions to identify what feels best for both partners, keeping the focus on comfort and consent to create a safe space. As you explore, you'll notice how the G-Spot not only adds to physical sensations but also deepens emotional bonds, paving the way for a more fulfilling and loving relationship.

Enhancing Intimacy through G-Spot Play

When it comes to deepening the connection between partners, G-Spot stimulation offers a unique and powerful pathway. The G-Spot, a sensitive and often elusive area, is much more than a physical structure; it serves as an intimate bridge, encouraging profound emotional and physical bonds between partners.

Exploring the G-Spot together demands openness and clear communication. It's not just a journey of physical exploration but also emotional vulnerability. Couples who embark on this exploration will find that the communication it requires can bring them closer, fostering a deep sense of trust and intimacy. Sharing intimate desires and boundaries openly creates a foundation for pleasurable experiences and intimate growth.

The initial steps in G-Spot play for couples often begin with exploration and learning. Taking the time to understand this sensitive area, locating it, and experimenting with different forms of touch can be both educational and erotic. Partners might start with gentle, exploratory touches, gradually increasing pressure and experimenting with varied techniques. This process allows for discovering what feels best for the receiving partner.

Creating a comfortable and inviting atmosphere enhances the experience. Soft lighting, soothing music, and warm, inviting settings can play a significant role in relaxing both partners. The mental state of each person can greatly influence physical pleasure, so prioritizing relaxation and comfort is crucial. A relaxed and open-minded attitude paves the way for more profound sensations and enjoyment.

Encouraging feedback during G-Spot play is essential. Partners should feel empowered to voice their preferences, dislikes, and intensity levels. Positive reinforcement and responsive adjustment to each other's cues enable a tailored experience, maximizing pleasure and connection.

Physical techniques are crucial in enhancing intimacy through G-Spot stimulation. Couples can explore different positions to find what works best for them. Positions that allow easy access and comfortable angles, such as the missionary or spooning positions, can facilitate more effective G-Spot stimulation. Experimenting with variations of these positions can offer different sensations and allow for deeper penetration and better access to the G-Spot.

Using toys specifically designed for G-Spot stimulation can also add variety and enhance pleasure. Curved dildos, vibrators, and other toys can provide targeted stimulation and introduce new sensations.

When introducing toys, it's important to maintain communication and reassure your partner that their comfort and enjoyment are paramount. Using toys should be a mutual decision, enhancing the collaborative nature of the experience.

Mutual trust and consent are the cornerstones of any intimate exploration. Boundaries should be established and respected. If discomfort or pain arises, it's important to stop immediately and address any concerns or adjustments needed. Honoring each other's limits ensures that the experience remains positive and enriching.

Couples who practice G-Spot play often report that it strengthens their relationship beyond the bedroom. The process of exploring and discovering each other's bodies can lead to increased intimacy, improved communication, and a deepened sense of partnership. The shared experiences contribute to a richer, more satisfying sexual relationship and can translate into a more profound emotional connection.

To truly enhance intimacy through G-Spot play, it's crucial to integrate it as part of a broader spectrum of sexual and emotional bonding. Combined with other intimate activities such as kissing, caressing, and verbal affirmations, G-Spot stimulation becomes a component of a holistic approach to deepening intimacy. Foreplay and aftercare, inclusive of gentle touches and affectionate gestures, play significant roles in framing the experience within a context of love and tenderness.

In conclusion, enhancing intimacy through G-Spot play is a multifaceted journey that involves physical discovery, emotional openness, and mutual respect. It provides a unique opportunity for couples to connect on a deeper level, building trust and enhancing their overall relationship. With clear communication, a comfortable setting, and a willingness to explore, couples can experience profound joy and closeness through G-Spot stimulation.

Communication and Positioning

In the journey of exploring G-spot stimulation as a couple, communication is your foundation. Honest and open dialogue sets the stage for experiences that are both pleasurable and deeply connecting. Start by discussing your desires, boundaries, and any past experiences that may inform your current approach. It can be as simple as sharing what you're curious about or as detailed as mapping out what kind of touch feels good. The key is to create a safe space where both partners feel heard and respected.

Before diving into the physical aspects, sit down together and have a candid conversation. Talk about what you're looking to get out of G-spot exploration. Are you aiming to deepen your intimacy, explore new forms of pleasure, or maybe both? Establishing mutual goals helps align your efforts and manage expectations. An open discussion about comfort levels, consent, and safe words is non-negotiable, allowing both of you to fully relax and enjoy the experience.

Remember, communication isn't a one-time event but an ongoing process. Check in with each other before, during, and after your sessions. Ask questions like, "How does this feel for you?" or "Would you like me to try something different?" Your partner's feedback is invaluable and will guide you in fine-tuning your technique for maximum pleasure.

Once you've established a strong foundation of communication, it's time to consider positioning. The right position can make all the difference in finding and stimulating the G-spot. Comfort is paramount, so think about what positions allow both of you to relax and maintain the kind of touch you're striving for.

One popular position for G-spot stimulation is the classic "missionary" with a twist. Elevate your partner's hips with a pillow—it helps angle the pelvis to allow for deeper penetration and easier access to the G-spot. This adjustment may seem minor, but it can significantly enhance the sensation for the receiving partner. Another versatile position is "doggy style," which provides deeper penetration and easier access to the G-spot from a different angle. Communication is key here; make sure your partner is comfortable with the depth and pace.

For couples who prefer face-to-face contact, the "spooning" position can be intimate and comfortable. This position allows for a gentle, controlled pace and the flexibility to make adjustments easily. It also offers the added benefit of being able to stimulate the clitoris simultaneously, which can result in blended orgasms—enhancing the overall experience.

Experimentation is part of the fun, so don't be afraid to try different angles and positions. You might discover that a subtle shift in your bodies makes a world of difference in the sensation. Your comfort and connection as a couple should guide your exploration, allowing you to find what feels best for both partners.

Using toys can also be an exciting way to explore G-spot stimulation. Communicate openly about which toys you'd like to incorporate and why. Both partners should feel comfortable and enthusiastic about the choices. Toys like G-spot vibrators or curved dildos can add a new dimension of pleasure and allow for precise stimulation. Discuss and decide together on the right time to introduce toys, and always prioritize comfort and consent.

Regardless of whether you're using toys or relying purely on manual techniques, rhythm and pressure play crucial roles in G-spot stimulation. Maintain a consistent yet adaptable approach—start with gentle pressure and gradually increase if it feels right. The optimal level of pressure varies from person to person, so ongoing communication during the act is essential. Encourage your partner to vocalize or use non-verbal cues to guide you.

After your exploration, take the time to debrief together. This post-play communication can be incredibly intimate and informative. Discuss what worked, what didn't, and how the experience made each of you feel. Feedback is a gift that can guide your future sessions and help you grow closer as a couple.

When both partners are engaged in this continuous loop of communication, it fosters a deeper emotional connection. You're not just sharing physical pleasure; you're sharing trust, vulnerability, and mutual respect. This connection extends beyond the bedroom and can strengthen your relationship in profound ways.

Remember, the ultimate goal is mutual pleasure and deeper intimacy. There's no rush or specific endpoint you need to reach. Enjoy the journey, celebrate the successes, and learn from the challenges. Your relationship's strength lies in how you communicate and navigate these intimate moments together, creating a more fulfilling connection both sexually and emotionally.

To sum up, the intersection of communication and positioning in G-spot stimulation is where physical pleasure meets emotional intimacy. By prioritizing honest dialogue, experimenting with positions, and remaining open to feedback, you and your partner can cultivate a richer, more fulfilling sexual relationship.

Chapter 13:
P-Spot Stimulation for Couples

Delving into P-Spot stimulation as a couple is a powerful way to deepen your emotional and physical connection. It involves more than just technique; it's about cultivating trust, curiosity, and candid communication with your partner. When you explore this intimate territory together, you're opening the door to new realms of pleasure and mutual understanding. Partnered P-Spot stimulation requires patience, a mindful approach, and an openness to experiment and share each other's boundaries and desires. With each touch and exploration, you're not only enhancing the sensory experience but also weaving a fabric of trust and closeness that strengthens your bond. Embrace the journey together, allowing it to enrich your intimate relationship in ways you might never have imagined.

Partnered Techniques

P-Spot stimulation, or prostate stimulation, can be a profoundly rewarding experience for couples who approach it with mutual trust and curiosity. It's more than just a physical act; it necessitates empathy, communication, and a willingness to explore each other's boundaries and desires. Understanding partnered techniques for P-Spot stimulation can enhance intimacy, bring about new levels of pleasure, and strengthen your connection.

Before diving into the specific techniques, it's crucial to create an environment where both partners feel safe and comfortable.

Discussing boundaries, likes, and dislikes beforehand can set the stage for a more open and enjoyable experience. Use this time to talk about what you're both interested in exploring and what you might want to avoid. Establish a safe word or signal to ensure that either partner can communicate discomfort or the need to stop at any time.

Preparation is key. Make sure that you're both relaxed and in the right mindset. Foreplay can be incredibly beneficial here, as it helps both partners to relax and become more attuned to each other's bodies. Engaging in mutual massage, deep kissing, or other forms of foreplay can help to eliminate any feelings of anxiety and make the experience more enjoyable for both partners.

One of the foundational techniques for partnered P-Spot stimulation involves manual exploration. Start by washing your hands and ensuring that your nails are trimmed and smooth to avoid any discomfort. Using plenty of water-based lubricant is essential for a comfortable and pleasurable experience. Encourage the receiving partner to find a position that feels relaxing and secure, such as lying on their back with their knees bent or on all fours.

Begin by gently massaging the area around the anus to help your partner relax. Slowly and carefully insert a lubricated finger, being mindful of your partner's comfort levels. Once inside, use a 'come-hither' motion to locate the P-Spot, which is typically found about two inches in along the front wall of the rectum. Communication is key during this process, so keep checking in with your partner to ensure that they are enjoying the sensations and feel comfortable.

Another effective technique involves incorporating toys designed for P-Spot stimulation. Toys such as prostate massagers can offer more consistent and targeted stimulation than manual techniques alone. When selecting a toy, look for ones that are specifically designed for prostate play, featuring a curved or angled shape that targets the P-Spot effectively. Always use plenty of lubricant and introduce the toy slowly, giving your partner time to adjust to the new sensation.

The use of a vibrating prostate massager can add an extra layer of stimulation. These devices often have multiple settings, allowing you to find the vibration intensity that works best for your partner. Experimenting with different rhythms and intensities can lead to a rich variety of pleasurable sensations. Just like with manual stimulation, communication is essential. Adjust based on your partner's feedback to ensure the experience remains pleasurable and comfortable.

P-Spot stimulation can also be combined with other forms of pleasure for an even more intense experience. Stimulating the penis or perineum simultaneously with P-Spot play can lead to powerful, blended orgasms. You can use your free hand, a toy, or even a vibrator to provide additional stimulation. Pay attention to how your partner reacts to different combinations and intensities of stimuli.

For many couples, incorporating P-Spot stimulation into their sexual routine can strengthen their emotional bond. The act of exploring a partner's body in such an intimate and vulnerable way requires a high degree of trust and open communication. These are the same elements that lay the foundation for a strong and healthy relationship. Take this opportunity to connect with your partner on a deeper emotional level.

Aftercare is an important part of the experience. After you finish, take time to cuddle, hold each other, and talk about what you both enjoyed. This can help to solidify the positive experience and leave both partners feeling satisfied and emotionally connected. Discussing what worked well and any areas of discomfort can also help to improve future experiences.

Keep in mind that not every session will go perfectly, and that's okay. The journey of exploring partnered P-Spot stimulation is about learning and growing together. Approach each experience with an open mind and a willingness to adapt. By continuously communicating and experimenting, you'll find what techniques work best for you as a couple.

Ultimately, the goal of partnered P-Spot stimulation techniques is to enhance the sexual pleasure and emotional intimacy between you and your partner. It's an ongoing journey of discovery and trust, one that can yield incredible rewards both in and out of the bedroom. So, take your time, communicate openly, and savor the journey together.

Building Trust and Connection

Trust and connection form the bedrock of any intimate relationship. When it comes to exploring P-Spot stimulation for couples, these elements become even more vital. P-Spot play requires a level of vulnerability and openness that many may find daunting at first, but the rewards—both emotional and physical—are well worth the effort. Simply put, building trust and connection is about creating a safe space where both partners feel comfortable exploring new realms of pleasure together.

First and foremost, open and honest communication sets the stage for successful P-Spot exploration. Discussing boundaries, expectations, and desires isn't just a preliminary step; it's an ongoing conversation. It's important to understand that people's comfort levels may change over time, and what's consensual and pleasurable one day might not be the next. By regularly checking in with each other, both partners can ensure that their experiences are enjoyable and pressure-free.

One practical way to build trust is through shared vulnerability. It's not uncommon for P-Spot stimulation to evoke a range of emotions, from intense pleasure to unexpected feelings of intimacy or even discomfort. When both partners are open about their experiences and emotions, they can offer each other the support needed to navigate these complex sensations. This mutual openness can deepen the emotional bond, turning P-Spot exploration into an act of trust-building rather than mere physical pleasure.

It's also helpful to establish a safe word or signal before diving into any form of P-Spot play. This ensures that either partner can halt the activity immediately if something feels off. Knowing that you have the power to stop can make it easier to relax and fully immerse in the experience, thereby fostering a sense of safety and security. This, in turn, can enhance the pleasure and emotional connection during P-Spot stimulation.

Creating a comfortable, inviting environment is another key aspect of building trust. Think about how you can set the mood: dim lighting, soft music, and perhaps aromatherapy can all contribute to a relaxing atmosphere that helps reduce anxiety. When the environment feels safe and inviting, it's easier to let go of reservations and focus on mutual pleasure. Make sure that all necessary items—such as lubrication and clean towels—are within easy reach to avoid any interruptions that might break the mood.

Patience is crucial. It's essential to proceed slowly and listen to each other's cues. This isn't just about physical readiness; it's about emotional readiness too. Sometimes, the body may not respond as quickly as hoped, but that's perfectly normal. The willingness to take time—to understand and respect each other's pace—demonstrates care and consideration, which strengthens the relationship.

Let's not forget the importance of aftercare. Aftercare involves taking the time to connect and communicate after the exploration is over. This could involve cuddling, talking about what you both enjoyed, and even discussing what could be improved for next time. Aftercare solidifies the bond of trust, reaffirming that the emotional connection is just as important as the physical one.

Now, let's talk about affirmations and positive reinforcement. Compliment each other not just on physical performance, but on the courage and trust displayed throughout the experience. Recognize and appreciate the efforts made by each partner to engage in this deeply personal form of intimacy. Positive reinforcement strengthens the connection and boosts confidence, making future P-Spot play even more enjoyable.

Building trust also means educating yourselves together. Read about P-Spot anatomy, techniques, and experiences from reliable sources. Watching educational videos or even attending workshops can provide a better understanding and build confidence. Sharing this learning journey not only increases knowledge but also cements a sense of partnership and mutual respect.

Incorporate playfulness into the experience. Humor can be a great way to alleviate any tension or awkwardness. A lighthearted approach can make the process enjoyable and less intimidating, thereby fostering a sense of ease and connection. Laughter, after all, is one of the best ways to build intimacy.

Mental and emotional preparedness play a noticeable role in how trust and connection evolve. Taking the time to meditate, practice mindfulness, or engage in other preparatory activities can help center both partners, making them more present for each other. The mental clarity achieved through such practices can create a more fulfilling and connected experience.

In conclusion, building trust and connection is not a one-time effort but an ongoing process. As you journey through P-Spot exploration together, remember that your emotional bond is the strongest tool in your arsenal. Open communication, shared vulnerability, patience, aftercare, and mutual respect will guide you in creating not just a pleasurable experience, but a deeply connected and trusting relationship. The investment you make in each other's comfort and joy will return to you tenfold, enriching your intimate lives in ways you perhaps never thought possible.

Chapter 14:
Combining G-Spot and
Clitoral Stimulation

Blending G-spot and clitoral stimulation can be a transformative experience, uniting profound internal pleasure with the external ecstasy of the clitoris. To achieve this harmonious balance, it's essential to communicate openly with your partner or to be attuned to your body's unique responses if exploring solo. Start with gentle, deliberate movements, both internally and externally, building a rhythm that feels intuitive. The synergy between G-spot and clitoral sensations can elevate arousal, often leading to powerful, blended orgasms that resonate on multiple levels. The key is to experiment and be patient, allowing your body's natural responses to guide the process. With practice and dedication, combining these techniques can deepen intimacy and greatly enhance overall pleasure.

Techniques for Blended Orgasms

Blending G-spot and clitoral stimulation can lead to intense and deeply satisfying orgasms. Combining these two powerful forms of stimulation isn't just about technique; it's also about understanding and tuning into your body's unique responses. This process requires patience, exploration, and open communication, whether you're engaging in solo play or partnered sessions.

One fundamental approach to achieving blended orgasms is synchronizing different types of touch. Begin by exploring the G-spot with gentle, rhythmic pressure using your fingers or a specially designed G-spot toy. At the same time, incorporate clitoral stimulation using light circular motions or a vibrating toy. The synchronization of internal and external sensations can create a powerful buildup of pleasure, leading to a more intense and fulfilling climax.

Timing plays an essential role in achieving a blended orgasm. It's not just about stimulating the G-spot and clitoris simultaneously; it's also about understanding when to increase or decrease the intensity of each type of stimulation. Listen to your body's signals. As arousal builds, you may find that alternating between G-spot and clitoral focus helps sustain pleasure and prevents overstimulation. The ebb and flow of sensation keep the experience dynamic and engaging.

Experimenting with different positions can also enhance your experience. For solo play, lying on your back with a pillow under your hips can elevate your pelvis, making it easier to reach and stimulate the G-spot while accessing the clitoris. For couples, positions like missionary or cowgirl can allow for simultaneous stimulation. In missionary, a toy or your partner's hand can focus on the G-spot while the clitoris is stimulated. In cowgirl, grinding against your partner's pelvis can provide clitoral stimulation while a finger or toy targets the G-spot.

Mindfulness and relaxation are equally important. The brain is a powerful organ in sexual response, and engaging in practices like deep breathing or meditation can help you stay present, reducing anxiety and enhancing pleasure. Let go of any preconceived notions about how the experience "should" unfold and embrace the authenticity of your sensations.

Communication is key when exploring blended orgasms with a partner. Clearly expressing your preferences and feedback ensures that your partner can make the right adjustments in real time. Remember, what feels incredible one day might be different the next. A shared journey of exploration can build intimacy and trust, making the experience more rewarding for both.

Introducing toys into your routine can also add a new dimension to blended stimulation. A dual-stimulation vibrator, designed to simultaneously target the G-spot and clitoris, can be a game-changer. Experiment with different settings and intensities to find what works best for you. For couples, experimenting with remote-controlled toys can add an element of surprise and control, creating a playful and intimate connection.

Lubrication is a critical component in achieving blended orgasms. Adequate lubrication ensures comfort and can enhance the sensations of both G-spot and clitoral stimulation. Invest in a high-quality, body-safe lubricant and apply it generously. Reapply as needed to maintain comfort and friction-free pleasure.

As you explore these techniques, it's essential to remain patient and compassionate with yourself. Sexual exploration is a journey, and what works may vary each time. Don't rush the process. Allow yourself to savor the journey and celebrate small victories along the way. Sometimes, the path to a blended orgasm can be just as fulfilling as the destination.

Lastly, consider the emotional context of your sexual experiences. Intimacy isn't solely about physical sensation; it's also about emotional closeness and connection. Cultivate an environment that feels safe, loving, and accepting. Emotional intimacy can enhance physical pleasure, making the experience of blended orgasms even more profound and fulfilling.

By combining G-spot and clitoral stimulation, you're opening the door to new dimensions of pleasure. The techniques outlined here serve as a guide to help you navigate this intricate dance. Remember, the most important aspect is to listen to your body, communicate openly with your partner, and prioritize pleasure and connection. With practice and patience, blended orgasms can become a meaningful part of your sexual repertoire, enriching your intimate experiences and deepening your connection with yourself and your partner.

Enhancing Overall Pleasure

When it comes to combining G-spot and clitoral stimulation, the opportunities for enhancing overall pleasure are immense and thrilling. This synergy can lead to what is often described as blended orgasms, where the sensations from both erogenous zones amplify and harmonize, creating a more profound and fulfilling experience. It's not just about achieving an orgasm; it's about exploring the depths of your sexual potential and enriching your intimate connections.

First, let's understand why combining these forms of stimulation can lead to such heightened pleasure. The G-spot, a sensitive area located within the front wall of the vagina, responds to firm, consistent pressure. Meanwhile, the clitoris, with its nerve-dense structure, reacts to lighter, rhythmic touches. When these stimulations occur simultaneously, they can create a pleasurable tension and a build-up of energy that cascades into a deeper release. This interplay of sensations can stimulate various pathways in the brain, leading to fuller and more satisfying orgasms.

One practical approach to enhancing overall pleasure is to alternate between focusing on the G-spot and clitoris. This can help in building anticipation and intensifying the sensations. For instance, start with gentle clitoral stimulation to awaken and arouse, then shift to more direct G-spot massage. As the intensity builds, alternating between the two can keep the excitement high and prevent numbing or overstimulation of either area.

For those experimenting with toys, dual-stimulation devices can be particularly effective. These toys are designed specifically to target both the G-spot and clitoris simultaneously, allowing for hands-free exploration that can lead to hands-free orgasms. In selecting such toys, it's crucial to consider size, shape, and vibration modes to find what feels most comfortable and pleasurable. Many find that a combination of pulsating vibrations for the clitoris and consistent pressure for the G-spot works wonders.

Couples can profoundly benefit from combining these techniques. For example, a partner can use their fingers or a toy to stimulate the G-spot while simultaneously using their tongue or another toy on the clitoris. Communication is vital here; verbal cues and body language can guide your partner in understanding which techniques work best and how to adjust pressure and speed. This shared journey becomes not just about reaching orgasm, but about deepening intimacy and trust.

Of course, the overall experience isn't just about physical techniques. The mind plays a significant role in sexual pleasure. Creating a relaxed and emotionally charged environment can greatly enhance the sensations from combined G-spot and clitoral stimulation. Set the scene with dim lighting, soft music, and perhaps even some scented candles to engage all your senses. The more comfortable and aroused you feel, the more your body will be responsive to the dual stimulation.

Additionally, experimenting with different positions can also enhance overall pleasure. Positions that allow easy access to both the G-spot and clitoris are ideal. For solo play, consider lying on your back with pillows supporting your lower back to increase the angle for G-spot access while using a hand or toy for clitoral stimulation. For couples, the missionary position can be adapted with the woman lying on her back and the man slightly tilted to be able to reach the G-spot with his fingers while thrusting. Adding a vibrator to the mix can elevate this experience even further.

Lastly, don't underestimate the power of mental focus and mindfulness. Concentrating on the sensations you're experiencing and letting go of distractions can significantly enhance your overall pleasure. Techniques like guided visualization or deep breathing can help you stay present and amplify your enjoyment. The concept of mindfulness in sex, often referred to as "mindful sex," encourages you to fully engage with the moment, increasing both physical and emotional satisfaction.

The journey to exquisite pleasure through combined G-spot and clitoral stimulation is unique to every individual and couple. It's a personal exploration that invites creativity, communication, and an open heart. The path might involve some trial and error, but with patience and a sense of adventure, the rewards are deeply fulfilling. Whether through solo exploration or shared moments with a partner, this combination offers limitless potential to enhance your sexual experience.

Chapter 15:
Combining P-Spot and
Penile Stimulation

Embarking on the journey to combine P-Spot and penile stimulation can unlock an enriched tapestry of sexual satisfaction and profound intimacy. This dual approach leverages the deeply sensitive prostate while simultaneously engaging the robust tactile pleasure of the penis, creating a symphony of sensations that resonate through the body. By carefully synchronizing rhythmic movements and pressure, either manually or with the aid of toys, you can explore the exquisite balance that maximizes pleasure. Communication with your partner, or mindful attunement during solo exploration, is key to ensuring comfort and elation, turning the experience into a deeply rewarding practice. As techniques are refined and mutual trust is deepened, the potential for immensely satisfying orgasms expands, offering a heightened sense of connection and fulfillment. This chapter is designed to guide you through the techniques and considerations for achieving this dual pleasure, making your intimate moments more exciting and deeply gratifying.

Techniques for Dual Pleasure

Exploring dual pleasure by combining P-Spot and penile stimulation offers a unique pathway to heightened sexual satisfaction. Delving into both realms concurrently can significantly enhance overall pleasure, fostering a deeper connection with one's partner or oneself. This approach encompasses a blend of manual techniques, the strategic use of sex toys, and understanding the synergy between these two pleasure zones.

Beginning with the manual techniques, it's critical to recognize the value of preparation and communication. For partnered activities, establishing trust and clearly expressing desires and boundaries is foundational. Both parties should feel comfortable and at ease, as this helps in creating a receptive environment for dual stimulation. For solo play, mental relaxation and a heightened state of arousal facilitate deeper exploration.

The process often starts with gradual, gentle stimulation, focusing on relaxation and increased blood flow to the pelvic region. Manual penile stimulation, such as light stroking or gentle squeezing, can be integrated with the rhythmic massaging of the P-Spot, using a well-lubricated finger to press and stroke in a slow, deliberate motion. The key here is synchronization. Finding a rhythm that harmoniously combines these actions can lead to intense pleasure and potentially powerful orgasms.

Moving on to toys, the modern world offers a variety of instruments designed to make blending P-Spot and penile stimulation seamless. Dual-action devices that cater specifically to these experiences can target both pleasure points simultaneously. For instance, certain prostate massagers come with external stimulators that can vibrate at various intensities, adding to the sensations experienced from P-Spot stimulation. Pairing these with a penis ring can keep the arousal levels high and potent.

Exploring multiple positions can amplify this experience. Positions that offer easy access to the P-Spot while allowing for manual or toy-assisted penile stimulation work best. Lying on one's back with legs lifted or pulling knees to the chest can provide optimal angles for dual stimulation. Partners might find success with one partner on top, manipulating both areas with ease, ensuring sustained contact and adjustable pressure.

Breathing techniques play a crucial role in maximizing dual pleasure. Deep, steady breathing helps distribute sensations throughout the body, increasing present awareness and enhancing the experience. Encourage partners to synchronize their breathing, fostering a deeper emotional and physical bond. This shared rhythm can amplify pleasure for both parties.

Mindfulness and conscious engagement can transform the experience from a simple act of pleasure to an enriching, intimate encounter. Being attuned to one's own bodily responses, as well as a partner's cues, cultivates a deeper sensory connection. This level of presence assists in identifying the exact moment when slight adjustments can propel pleasure to its peak. Establishing eye contact and verbal affirmations during the process can further deepen intimacy and increase mutual satisfaction.

Additionally, alternating between techniques and sensations keeps the experience dynamic and captivating. Shifting from gentle to firm pressure, or fluctuating the speed and rhythm of stimulation, can prevent desensitization and keep the pleasure at its apex. Variety fosters a sense of anticipation and continuous engagement, making each session unique and exciting.

Combining P-Spot and penile stimulation is not solely about physical acts; it's an encounter enriched with emotional intimacy and mutual exploration. Engage in discussions about what feels good, share fantasies, and remain open to experimenting with new techniques. Communication is fundamental, whether that's through verbal cues, body language, or expressions of pleasure and consent.

Finally, post-encounter care is as important as the experience itself. Aftercare involving intimate touch, affirmations, and shared relaxation fosters a sense of safety and deep connection. Reflecting on the experience together, discussing what worked well and what could be tweaked, encourages a continuous journey of discovery and mutual satisfaction.

Achieving dual pleasure through the simultaneous engagement of the P-Spot and penile stimulation offers a profound path to enhanced intimacy and orgasmic satisfaction. It requires a balance of careful technique, mindful presence, and open communication. When approached with care and creativity, this practice can elevate the sexual experience to new, unexplored dimensions.

Maximizing Sexual Satisfaction

Combining P-Spot and penile stimulation offers a unique and deeply satisfying experience for those who are willing to explore and experiment. The key lies in understanding the synergy between these two powerful forms of pleasure. Both the P-Spot and the penis provide intense, yet distinct sensations. When stimulated together, they can amplify each other, creating waves of ecstasy that ripple through the entire body.

The art of maximizing sexual satisfaction with this dual approach requires open communication, patience, and a willingness to explore. Whether you are exploring solo or with a partner, starting with a relaxed and open mindset is crucial. Take time to understand your body or your partner's body, preferences, and comfort levels. Establishing a safe and comfortable environment will help to facilitate deeper levels of pleasure and connection.

Positioning plays a vital role in combining P-Spot and penile stimulation. Each person's anatomy is unique, and finding the right angle and method may require some trial and error. Experiment with different positions to discover what feels best. For instance, the "cowboy" or "reverse cowboy" position can offer direct stimulation to the P-Spot while allowing for various angles of penile pleasure. Likewise, positions that involve lifting the hips or using pillows for support can make both forms of stimulation more accessible and enjoyable.

When engaging in combined stimulation, it is essential to be mindful of rhythm and pressure. Some may prefer gentle, consistent pressure on the P-Spot while varying the speed and technique of penile stimulation. Others may enjoy alternating between intense, focused stimulation and softer, more diffuse touches. Communication, whether verbal or non-verbal, will help guide the experience and ensure both parties are fully attuned to each other's needs and desires.

Lubrication is another critical component in achieving maximum satisfaction. The anus does not naturally produce lubrication, so using a good quality, body-safe lubricant is essential to reduce friction and enhance comfort. Choosing the right lubricant can make a significant difference; water-based lubricants are versatile and suitable for most toys, while silicone-based lubricants provide longer-lasting slickness.

Incorporating toys can further enhance the experience of combining P-Spot and penile stimulation. Prostate massagers, vibrating anal beads, and dual stimulation toys are designed to target the P-Spot with precision, while still allowing for hand or oral stimulation of the penis. High-quality, well-designed toys can heighten sensations and add a new dimension to the experience.

Breathwork and relaxation techniques can significantly enhance the experience. Controlling your breathing helps maintain a connection to the body and the sensations being experienced. Deep, rhythmic breathing can also intensify orgasms and help sustain arousal for longer periods. Practice mindfulness, staying present in the moment, and focusing on the pleasures coursing through your body. This can amplify both physical and emotional satisfaction.

Building sexual satisfaction is not just about the physical aspects but also emotional intimacy. Sharing this experience can deepen your connection with your partner, creating a bond that goes beyond the physical. Take time before, during, and after to connect, share feelings, and reflect on the experience. Such openness and vulnerability can foster trust and intimacy, enriching your relationship and sexual experiences further.

Additionally, consider incorporating elements of eroticism and fantasy to keep the experience exciting and fresh. Discuss fantasies and desires with your partner, and explore role-playing or other forms of erotic exploration. Allowing yourselves to be creative and adventurous can lead to new discoveries and a deeper understanding of each other's pleasures.

Post-play aftercare is just as important as the play itself. Spend time together winding down, cuddling, and talking about the experience. This aftercare helps in integrating the physical sensations with emotional connections, ensuring that both partners feel valued and cared for. It fosters a sense of closeness and satisfaction that lingers long after the physical sensations have subsided.

In conclusion, the journey of maximizing sexual satisfaction through combining P-Spot and penile stimulation is a deeply personal and rewarding one. It requires intention, communication, and a willingness to explore uncharted territories of pleasure. By integrating these practices into your intimate life, you can unlock new realms of ecstasy and deepen both physical and emotional connections.

Remember, sexual satisfaction is a dynamic and evolving experience. Stay curious, and don't be afraid to try new things and revisit old favorites. The more you understand and appreciate the intricate dance between the P-Spot and penile stimulation, the more profound and fulfilling your intimate moments will be. Enjoy the journey and embrace the boundless possibilities of pleasure.

Chapter 16:
Safety and Hygiene for
G-Spot Stimulation

Ensuring safety and maintaining proper hygiene during G-Spot stimulation is essential for a pleasurable and healthy experience. Begin by washing your hands thoroughly and cleaning under your nails to prevent the spread of bacteria. Using a high-quality, water-based lubricant can enhance comfort and reduce friction, which is particularly important since the vaginal tissues are sensitive. Make sure to clean any toys thoroughly before and after use, following the manufacturer's guidelines—typically involving mild soap and warm water. Consider using condoms or toy covers for added cleanliness, especially if you're sharing toys. Lastly, listen to your body and never force any activity that causes pain or discomfort. By prioritizing cleanliness and safety, you can ensure that your experiences are both enjoyable and worry-free.

Best Practices for Cleanliness

Ensuring cleanliness is paramount when engaging in G-spot stimulation. Good hygiene not only fosters a healthy and safe environment but can also enhance the overall experience, making it more enjoyable and worry-free. The aim here is to understand and embrace these practices to set the stage for intimate exploration with confidence.

Before diving into the mechanics, the first step in cleanliness is hand hygiene. Always start by thoroughly washing your hands with warm water and soap. It may seem basic, but clean hands can prevent the introduction of bacteria and help avoid potential infections. Consider trimming and filing your fingernails to avoid any accidental scratches or discomfort during exploration.

Next, let's discuss the tools and toys used for G-spot stimulation. Whether you're using your fingers, a specially designed toy, or a combination of both, cleanliness is crucial. If you're using toys, wash them before and after each use with mild soap and water or a toy cleaner. Always check the manufacturer's guidelines for care and maintenance to ensure the longevity and safety of your tools.

Using a condom over toys can add an extra layer of cleanliness, especially if sharing toys between partners or orifices. Condoms can help prevent the spread of bacteria and are easy to change between uses, making them a convenient option for maintaining hygiene.

Lubricants play a significant role in G-spot stimulation. They not only enhance pleasure but also reduce the risk of friction and discomfort. However, not all lubricants are created equal. Opt for water-based or silicone-based lubricants that are free from harmful chemicals and fragrances. Reapply as needed to maintain a smooth and pleasurable experience.

Speaking of lubricants, it's essential to keep them stored properly. Ensure they are kept in a cool, dry place, tightly sealed, and away from direct sunlight. Expired lubricants should be discarded, as they can lose their efficacy and may harbor bacteria. Always check the expiration date before using any product.

Positioning is another element to consider for cleanliness. A clean environment, such as a freshly laundered towel or sheet, can make a significant difference. This not only creates a hygienic space but also makes cleanup easier afterward. Consider having tissues or wet wipes on hand for any immediate needs.

For those who are menstruating, vaginal hygiene becomes even more critical. Some may feel comfortable exploring during their period, while others might prefer to wait. If you choose to engage in G-spot stimulation during menstruation, using a menstrual cup can help minimize mess and keep the area cleaner. Remember to clean the cup thoroughly according to the manufacturer's guidelines before and after use.

Communication between partners can't be overstated. Openly discussing cleanliness, boundaries, and comfort levels can build trust and ensure that both parties feel safe and respected. This dialogue can also cover any allergies or sensitivities either partner may have to certain products or materials.

Another often overlooked aspect is post-play hygiene. After any session of G-spot stimulation, it's essential to clean up properly. Urinating after sexual activity can help flush out any bacteria that may have entered the urethra, reducing the risk of urinary tract infections. Take the time to wash the genital area with warm water and a gentle, unscented soap to remove any lubricant or bodily fluids.

Nurturing a routine for cleanliness can become a seamless part of your personal and partnered practices. As with any aspect of intimate exploration, the more attuned you are to these practices, the more they become second nature, allowing you to focus solely on the joy and connection of the experience.

Lastly, consider the mental aspect of cleanliness. Feeling secure in your hygiene practices can alleviate anxiety and help you stay present. A clear, relaxed mind contributes to a more fulfilling and pleasurable experience, aligning body and spirit in the dance of intimate discovery.

In summary, maintaining cleanliness isn't just about physical steps; it's also about fostering a mindset of care and respect—for yourself and your partner. By adopting these best practices, you're crafting a safe, inviting, and pleasurable environment conducive to exploring the rich and rewarding world of G-spot stimulation.

Common Safety Concerns

When it comes to G-spot stimulation, safety and hygiene are paramount. While exploring this unique area can be immensely rewarding, it's essential to understand the potential risks and how to mitigate them effectively. Awareness and preparation can prevent discomfort, infections, and injuries, ensuring that the experience remains pleasurable and safe.

The first consideration is personal hygiene. Before engaging in any form of G-spot stimulation, ensure that both partners have clean hands. Thoroughly wash hands with soap and water to minimize the risk of introducing bacteria into the vaginal canal. This step is crucial, as the vagina is a delicate environment that can easily become unbalanced.

Trimmed nails are another small but significant detail. Sharp or jagged nails can cause micro-abrasions in the vaginal walls, leading to discomfort and potential infection. Investing in a good nail file and taking a few minutes to smooth out any rough edges can make a big difference. Additionally, consider wearing nitrile or latex gloves; they offer an extra layer of protection and are particularly useful if either partner has long nails.

It's also essential to use a high-quality, body-safe lubricant. The vaginal area does not always produce sufficient natural lubrication, especially during initial stages of arousal. A good lubricant reduces friction, preventing irritation and making the experience more enjoyable. Opt for water-based lubricants, as they are generally safe and compatible with most toys and condoms.

Speaking of toys, using products made from body-safe materials is non-negotiable. Silicone, glass, and stainless steel are excellent choices because they are non-porous and easy to clean. Avoid toys made from jelly or rubber, as these materials can harbor bacteria even after cleaning. Always clean toys before and after each use with an appropriate cleaner to maintain optimal hygiene.

Another crucial aspect is understanding the limits of pain and pleasure. Listen to your body and communicate openly with your partner. The thin line between discomfort and pleasure can sometimes be blurred, but the key is to avoid pushing beyond your comfort zone. If you experience pain, stop immediately and reassess the situation. Pain is your body's way of indicating that something isn't right.

Mindfulness about potential allergic reactions is also critical. Some individuals are sensitive to certain types of lubricants or materials used in sex toys. Test new products on a small area of your skin or use hypoallergenic products to avoid any adverse reactions. The last thing you want is to deal with itching or irritation during such an intimate moment.

For those using toys for G-spot stimulation, be cautious about the design and functionality. Avoid products with complex shapes or rough textures if you are new to this type of play. Simpler designs are easier to handle and clean, reducing the risk of injury and bacterial growth. Read reviews and choose well-regarded products from reputable brands.

Storage of your sexual wellness items also warrants attention. Keep toys in a cool, dry place away from direct sunlight. Many products come with their own storage pouches, which are ideal for maintaining cleanliness. Regularly inspect your toys for any signs of wear and tear;

damaged toys should be replaced immediately to avoid potential injuries.

Always use a condom on any toy that will be used internally, especially if sharing between partners. This practice not only maintains hygiene but also reduces the risk of sexually transmitted infections (STIs). Condoms create an additional barrier, adding an extra layer of safety to your intimacy.

Lastly, it's important to be aware of any medical conditions that could be exacerbated by G-spot stimulation. Conditions such as pelvic inflammatory disease (PID), vaginismus, or recent surgeries require careful consideration and perhaps even consultation with a healthcare provider before engaging in G-spot play. In such cases, professional advice can offer personalized recommendations to ensure a safe experience.

In conclusion, while G-spot stimulation can be an exciting and rewarding journey of sexual discovery, understanding common safety concerns and taking proactive measures can ensure that the experience is both safe and pleasurable. Prioritize hygiene, use body-safe materials, and communicate openly with your partner. Your journey into G-spot stimulation will be all the more enriching when approached with care and mindfulness.

Chapter 17:
Safety and Hygiene for
P-Spot Stimulation

When it comes to exploring P-Spot stimulation, safety and hygiene are paramount to ensuring a pleasurable and comfortable experience. Essential hygiene tips begin with thorough cleansing of hands and any toys that will be used. Use warm water and antimicrobial soap to help prevent infections. Similarly, communication is key; discussing comfort levels and boundaries with your partner can prevent misunderstandings and accidents. Lubrication is crucial in P-Spot stimulation to avoid any potential discomfort or tearing; opt for high-quality, water-based lubricants. After care should also not be neglected; a gentle rinse and reassuring words can make the entire experience feel more intimate and enjoyable. By prioritizing hygiene and safety, you lay a strong foundation for both physical and emotional enjoyment.

Essential Hygiene Tips

When exploring the deeply fulfilling realm of P-Spot stimulation, maintaining proper hygiene is of utmost importance. Not only does it enhance the overall experience, but it also ensures safety and comfort for both you and your partner. Hygiene isn't just about cleanliness; it's about creating an inviting, safe space free from potential infections or discomfort.

The anus and rectum can harbor bacteria, and using clean tools and techniques helps minimize risks. Before diving into P-Spot exploration, prepare with a few key practices. First and foremost, thoroughly wash your hands. This simple step is often underestimated but incredibly powerful in preventing the introduction of bacteria.

Next, consider the toys or objects you plan to use in your exploration. They must be either disposable or made from non-porous materials such as silicone, glass, or stainless steel. These materials are easier to clean and less likely to harbor bacteria. Make sure each toy is cleaned before and after use with warm water and mild soap or a dedicated toy cleaner. Avoid sharing toys, but if you must, use a condom as a barrier to add an extra layer of safety.

Speaking of condoms, their use isn't limited to penile or vaginal intercourse. Condoms can effectively cover toys or fingers used for P-Spot stimulation. They help keep everything clean, allowing both of you to fully immerse in the moment without anxiety about hygiene.

Another essential aspect is lubrication. The anus doesn't lubricate itself naturally, so generous use of a high-quality, body-safe lubricant is crucial. It reduces friction, which can tear the delicate tissue and create micro-abrasions that might become breeding grounds for bacteria. When selecting a lubricant, opt for water-based or silicone-based options. Oil-based lubricants can degrade the material of some toys and condoms, which is something to bear in mind.

For those integrating P-Spot play into their regular routine, more advanced preparations might become necessary. Some individuals choose to engage in a rectal cleansing (commonly known as an enema) prior to P-Spot stimulation. While not mandatory, it's a step that can enhance comfort and confidence. If you decide to use an enema, use warm water and be gentle to avoid irritation or damage to the sensitive anal tissue. Pay attention to your body's signals and stop if you experience discomfort.

It's also beneficial to trim and file any fingernails if they're part of your P-Spot exploration toolbox. Sharp or jagged edges can cause unintended scratches or discomfort. A pair of clean, trimmed, and filed nails shows care and consideration toward your or your partner's experience. Donning a latex or nitrile glove can provide an additional barrier, promoting cleanliness and reducing the risk of transferring bacteria.

Creating an environment where hygiene is a priority not only reduces physical risks but also fosters a trusting and relaxed atmosphere. Open communication with your partner about all facets of the experience, including hygiene, strengthens the emotional connection and paves the way for a more enjoyable journey. If you're practicing solo, incorporating these hygiene tips adds an extra layer of care and respect for yourself and your body.

Remember to account for aftercare, a crucial part of the hygienic process. Once the intimate session has concluded, both you and your partner should take a moment to clean up. This involves both washing the genital and anal areas to remove any lubricant, sweat, or other bodily fluids. A gentle wash with warm water and mild, unscented soap is best to avoid irritation. Ensure everything used during the session, including sheets or towels, gets cleaned to prevent any potential infections or unpleasant odors.

Finally, consider your overall health routine. Maintaining a balanced diet and staying hydrated promotes a healthier digestive system, contributing to the overall cleanliness and ease of P-Spot play. Regular exercise and good mental well-being also support your journey in exploring your sexuality. Staying informed and taking a holistic approach ensures that hygiene becomes an integral and effortless part of P-Spot stimulation.

As you navigate the intricate landscape of pleasure, the strategic steps you take to ensure cleanliness can amplify the joy, connection, and satisfaction you derive from P-Spot stimulation. By incorporating these essential hygiene tips into your practice, you create a safe, respectful, and deeply intimate experience that celebrates both the body and the spirit.

Addressing Safety Questions

When it comes to P-spot stimulation, safety is often the first concern for many individuals and couples. It's completely natural to have questions, and seeking answers is a wise step toward enhancing your intimate experiences safely. Let's unravel some of the most pressing safety issues and provide practical, science-backed solutions.

One of the primary concerns for many is the potential for injury. The prostate is a sensitive gland, and while it can deliver immense pleasure, it's crucial to approach stimulation with care. Using too much force or neglecting to communicate can lead to discomfort or even minor injuries. Always start slowly, using ample lubrication. Silicone-based lube tends to last longer and can make the experience much smoother. Additionally, attentive communication with your partner can ensure both parties remain comfortable and enjoy the experience.

Another common question revolves around the risk of infections. Since the P-spot is accessed via the anus, maintaining hygiene is non-negotiable. Before engaging in any play, ensure that both the anus and the surrounding area are thoroughly cleaned. Using an anal douche can be a helpful step for those particularly concerned about cleanliness. Make sure to clean any toys before and after use with antibacterial soap or a toy-specific cleaner to reduce the risk of infection.

Some worry about the introduction of bacteria from the anus into the urethra, especially when using prostate massagers or fingers. This concern can be mitigated by using condoms on toys or fingers, changing condoms when switching between different areas of the body, and through thorough hand washing. These practices contribute significantly to preventing infections and make the experience more comfortable for all involved.

For individuals new to P-spot stimulation, the idea of inserting objects into the anus can be unsettling due to the fear of losing them internally. To address this, always choose toys with a flared base or handle. This design prevents the toy from being fully inserted, providing a safe and worry-free experience. Additionally, opting for toys made from body-safe materials such as silicone, stainless steel, or glass can also minimize health risks.

Lubrication cannot be stressed enough. The anus does not produce natural lubrication, unlike the vaginal area. Using insufficient lube can lead to uncomfortable friction and potential microtears, increasing the risk of infections and other complications. Generously applying a high-quality lubricant can make a world of difference in ensuring a pleasurable and safe experience.

Mental comfort is another vital aspect. It's normal to experience a degree of anxiety or hesitation when exploring new facets of sexual pleasure. Communication and trust between partners can alleviate much of this apprehension. Discussing boundaries, safe words, and preferences before beginning can foster a more relaxed environment. Remember, all exploration should be enthusiastic and consensual.

The risk of overstimulation is worth noting. The P-spot, when stimulated, can produce intense sensations. While these can be thrilling, overdoing it can lead to sensitivity or even discomfort afterward. Moderation is key. Pay attention to your body's signals and take breaks as needed. Including periods of rest ensures that each session is not only enjoyable but also sustainable for future exploration.

It's important to be aware of your body's normal responses and understand what's typical for you. Any unusual pain, prolonged discomfort, or bleeding should not be ignored. In such cases, it's advisable to stop the activity and consult a healthcare provider. Proactive monitoring can help address potential issues before they escalate.

Sexual health practitioners frequently emphasize the importance of getting regular check-ups, especially for those active in anal play. These visits can help catch any infections or conditions early and provide peace of mind. Don't hesitate to bring up P-spot stimulation during your consultation—a knowledgeable professional can offer additional personalized advice and reassurance.

For those with specific medical conditions, such as hemorrhoids or anal fissures, it's crucial to consult a doctor before attempting P-spot stimulation. These conditions can complicate the process and lead to more severe health issues if not managed properly. Your doctor can provide guidance tailored to your situation and suggest safe ways to enjoy P-spot stimulation.

A final consideration is the psychological and emotional aspects of engaging in P-spot stimulation. Feelings of shame or embarrassment, often tied to cultural taboos, can impede the experience. Recognizing and addressing these emotions is essential. Educational resources, supportive communities, and open dialogues with partners can help dismantle these barriers, allowing a more fulfilling and positive exploration.

Chapter 18:
Overcoming Common Challenges
with G-Spot Stimulation

When exploring G-Spot stimulation, it's normal to encounter a few hurdles, but understanding how to navigate them can turn potential frustration into profound pleasure. Discomfort may arise from factors such as improper technique, tension, or even emotional barriers. To alleviate this, start with thorough communication, both with your partner and your own body. Ensure relaxation is at the forefront—use deep breathing and create a comfortable environment. Varying pressure and angles can also make a significant difference; sometimes, it's about discovering the right nuance that transforms discomfort into delight. Enhancing pleasure involves a combination of patience, gentle exploration, and attentiveness to what feels right in the moment. By prioritizing mindfulness and tenderness, the journey to G-Spot bliss becomes a more rewarding and less daunting experience.

Addressing Discomfort

It's not uncommon to feel some level of discomfort when exploring G-Spot stimulation. For many, this journey may involve physical and emotional hurdles. Understanding the nature of this discomfort is crucial. It can arise from a variety of factors, such as a lack of proper arousal, insufficient lubrication, or simply unfamiliarity with the sensations being experienced.

One of the most immediate causes of discomfort can be inadequate lubrication. The vagina is a dynamic, self-regulating ecosystem, and its natural lubrication levels can vary based on hormonal cycles, stress, and hydration. Using a high-quality, body-safe lubricant is essential. Lubricants can enhance sensations and reduce the friction that often causes discomfort. For those who are sensitive to certain ingredients, look for lubricants that are free from glycerin and parabens.

Another common factor is not being fully relaxed. Relaxation is key because muscle tension in the pelvic area can make G-Spot stimulation uncomfortable. Prioritize creating a relaxing environment. Consider dim lighting, soothing music, and perhaps a warm bath beforehand to help you unwind. Breathing exercises can also be invaluable. Deep, diaphragmatic breathing helps to relax the muscles of the pelvic floor and promote a state of relaxation throughout the body.

Let's address positioning. Certain sexual positions make it easier to access the G-Spot while minimizing discomfort. For solo play, lying on your back with your knees bent and legs apart can provide comfort and control. When with a partner, consider trying positions where you can control the depth and pace, like the cowgirl position. Clear communication with your partner is vital; let them know what feels good and what does not.

Emotional readiness is another layer that's often overlooked. Past experiences, societal conditioning, and personal insecurities can create mental blocks. It's essential to approach G-Spot exploration with a positive and open mindset. Patience with oneself and any partners involved can open the door to more fulfilling experiences. Establishing trust and open communication can ease these emotional barriers significantly.

Some individuals experience discomfort due to an overstimulation of the bladder, given the proximity of the G-Spot to the bladder. It's normal to feel the urge to urinate initially. This is because the G-Spot is located just behind the pubic bone, near the front wall of the vagina, so it can press against the bladder. It can be reassuring to empty your bladder before starting exploration. With continued stimulation, the urge typically reduces, revealing deeper layers of pleasure.

Discomfort can also be a sign that more arousal time is needed before attempting G-Spot stimulation. Foreplay is not just a precursor to the main event; it is an essential part of the experience. Engaging in extended foreplay ensures the body is sufficiently aroused, which allows for more comfortable and pleasurable G-Spot stimulation.

Mindful touch is another significant aspect that can help reduce discomfort. Slow, deliberate movements help in recognizing what feels good and what doesn't. Avoid rushing the process. Spend time exploring the sensations at different angles and pressures. A gentle "come hither" motion is often effective, but it's crucial to adjust based on feedback from your body or your partner's responses.

It's also important to recognize that everyone's anatomy is different. What works for one person may not work for another. This individuality means that some exploration and experimentation are necessary to find what is most pleasurable and least uncomfortable.

If you ever encounter persistent pain or significant discomfort, it might be time to consult a healthcare provider. There could be underlying medical conditions contributing to the discomfort. Healthcare providers specializing in sexual health can offer valuable insights and solutions that are tailored to individual needs.

Lastly, consider integrating feedback loops into the experience. Continuous communication with yourself or your partner about what feels good—and what doesn't—can significantly enhance the experience. Creating an open dialogue helps in making real-time adjustments that can mitigate discomfort and heighten pleasure.

Addressing discomfort in G-Spot stimulation is about combining practical steps with emotional preparedness. It's about creating an environment that fosters relaxation, using appropriate tools like high-quality lubricants, and maintaining a mindset that embraces exploration and patience. The journey to sexual pleasure is deeply personal and multifaceted, but with the right approach, the rewards can be profoundly fulfilling.

As you continue to explore, remember that discomfort does not have to be a barrier. It can be a signal and a guide, pushing you towards better understanding and more pleasurable experiences. Listen to your body, communicate openly with partners, and give yourself permission to discover what truly brings you joy.

Enhancing Pleasure

When aiming to enhance pleasure through G-spot stimulation, there's an exciting world of techniques and approaches to explore. Let's dive into some methods that will not only heighten your sensations but also deepen your emotional and physical connection, whether you're engaging in solo play or as a couple.

Understanding and bringing awareness to your body is fundamental. The way you perceive your own anatomy can significantly influence the depth of pleasure you experience. A crucial aspect of enhancing G-spot stimulation is nurturing a mindset of exploration and openness. This involves being mindful and present, tuning into the subtle cues of your body's responses, and allowing yourself to be immersed in the sensations.

It begins with being at ease. Relaxation goes a long way in enhancing pleasure. If tension is present, it can act as a barrier, preventing you from fully experiencing the wonders of G-spot stimulation. Create an environment where you feel completely comfortable and safe. Dim lighting, soft music, and perhaps soothing aromatherapy can set the mood and help you relax.

Incorporating mindfulness practices can further relax the body and mind. Deep breathing exercises, where you focus on each inhale and exhale, can center your attention on the present moment, stripping away distractions. Visualization techniques, where you imagine sensations like waves building and receding or a blooming flower, can enhance the overall experience by engaging your mind and body simultaneously.

Communication remains key, particularly in partnered scenarios. Discuss what feels good, what doesn't, and any adjustments needed to optimize the experience. Trust and openness with your partner create a secure environment where experimental techniques can be explored freely, fostering mutual pleasure. It's about co-creating a shared experience where both partners' desires and boundaries are respected and celebrated.

Variety in technique can also elevate your G-spot exploration. Manual stimulation, through varied pressure and movements, can uncover new pleasurable spots and sensations. Experimenting with different types of touch—light tapping, circular motions, or deeper, more consistent pressure—can reveal what feels most pleasurable. G-spot toys, specifically designed to target this erogenous zone, can add exciting dimensions to your play. Their contours and vibrations can offer new levels of stimulation that hands alone might not achieve.

An important yet often overlooked element is lubrication. A well-lubricated experience can minimize any discomfort and enhance sensitivity. High-quality, water-based lubricants are usually recommended for G-spot play, as they maintain moisture and reduce friction. Always ensure that the lubricant is compatible with any toys you might use to avoid damage and maintain optimal safety.

Temperature play can be an unexpected but delightful enhancement. Using warmed or cooled toys, or simply altering the temperature of your lubricant, can introduce new and exciting sensations. This element of surprise adds a thrilling layer to the experience, keeping it fresh and invigorating.

Exploring different positions can also bring about heightened pleasure. For instance, positions where the angle of penetration is more direct can intensify G-spot stimulation. Experiment with adjustments to conventional positions as well as trying out new ones to find what works best for you. Each body is unique, so the journey to discovering the most pleasurable positions can be a fun and intimate adventure in itself.

Additionally, combining G-spot stimulation with other types of erogenous zone activation can result in overwhelming and deeply satisfying orgasms. As noted in other sections of this book, stimulating the clitoris alongside the G-spot can create what some describe as a "blended orgasm," where the wealth of sensations comes together for a more profound and intense climax.

It's essential to give yourself permission to explore without judgment. Sexual exploration should be a liberating experience, unencumbered by societal pressures or personal insecurities. Embrace your desires and the wonderful complexities of your body's responses. It's not about chasing a specific outcome but rather enjoying the journey and the myriad sensations along the way.

To sum up, enhancing pleasure through G-spot stimulation is a multifaceted endeavor. It involves physical techniques, mental preparedness, and emotional openness. Whether you're delving into this solo or with a partner, the ultimate goal is a richer, more fulfilling sexual experience, grounded in knowledge, mutual respect, and a joyful curiosity. Let every encounter be an opportunity to learn more about yourself and discover new heights of pleasure.

Chapter 19:
Overcoming Common Challenges
with P-Spot Stimulation

Navigating the world of P-Spot stimulation can be both exciting and daunting, particularly when faced with common challenges such as heightened sensitivity and discomfort. First, recognize that sensitivity in this area is normal and can be managed with proper communication and technique. Initiate exploration with gentle pressure, experimenting with different angles and motions. Adding plenty of lubrication can significantly enhance comfort, minimizing friction and making the experience more pleasurable. It's also crucial to establish a relaxed environment, both mentally and physically, by engaging in deep breathing or a gentle massage beforehand. In cases where discomfort persists, don't hesitate to pause and revisit the techniques, making sure to listen to both your body and your partner's feedback. Overcoming these hurdles can lead to deeply fulfilling experiences, fostering a stronger, intimate connection and greater sexual satisfaction.

Dealing with Sensitivity

When it comes to P-Spot stimulation, sensitivity is a multifaceted subject that requires both awareness and finesse. Navigating the intricate tapestry of physical sensations is key to transforming P-Spot exploration from a curiosity into a profoundly enriching experience. Sensitivity in this context can span from slight pleasurable tinglings to intense, almost overwhelming feelings. Understanding how to manage and harness this sensitivity can make all the difference.

Not every experience of P-Spot stimulation will be the same, and acknowledging this variability helps set realistic expectations. There are days when sensitivity might be heightened due to various factors like stress, hydration, or even diet. On other days, the sensations might feel muted. Recognizing these fluctuations as normal can alleviate pressure to achieve a specific outcome every time.

One of the first steps in dealing with P-Spot sensitivity is listening to your body. Establish a rhythm with deep, relaxed breathing, allowing the body to signal its readiness. Timing plays a crucial role; sometimes, the body isn't prepared for such focused stimulation right away. In these cases, building anticipation through gentle caresses or external anal massage can be more beneficial than diving straight into deeper sensations.

Overcoming initial sensitivity often involves using lubrication generously. The rectal tissues are delicate and lack natural lubrication, making high-quality, body-safe lubricants indispensable. Silicone-based lubricants are a popular choice for their lasting slickness, although water-based options are easier to clean. Experimentation will reveal which type suits your body best. Don't hesitate to reapply as needed; when it comes to comfort, more is often better.

Desensitizing sprays and creams are another avenue for those experiencing extreme sensitivity. While these can be highly effective, use them sparingly. Overuse can dull sensations to the point where the experience loses its pleasure. Always start with the minimum amount to gauge your individual reaction. Remember, the goal is not to eradicate sensitivity but to bring it down to a manageable level.

Another vital aspect is mindfulness in touch. Gentle, consistent pressure is often more effective than hasty or erratic movements. Start with just a finger or a very slim toy to gauge the initial reactions. Over time, as the body becomes more accustomed, you can graduate to more substantial forms of stimulation. Communicate openly with your partner if you're in a shared experience. Their understanding and responsive touch can make navigating sensitivity a shared, intimate journey.

Varied techniques can also play a part in managing sensitivity. For instance, focusing on the area around the P-Spot rather than direct stimulation can significantly enhance comfort levels. Circular motions or shallow thrusts can offer ample pleasure without overwhelming initial sensitivity. Pull back and let the sensations build gradually rather than rushing toward a climax. This practice not only enhances enjoyment but also cultivates a deeper connection to your body's unique responses.

When sensitivity presents as discomfort or pain rather than pleasure, it's essential to pause and reassess. Pain is the body's way of signaling that something isn't right. This could be due to insufficient lubrication, positioning, or even a need for more relaxation. In such cases, adopting different positions can alleviate strain. For example, lying on your side with knees slightly drawn up might provide better access and reduce discomfort.

Communication, particularly with a partner, is critical. Expressing your comfort levels, needs, and boundaries fosters a safer, more relaxed environment. This open dialogue allows for real-time adjustments to techniques and pressure, enhancing the overall experience. Trust and patience from both partners can transform hesitant exploration into a deeply fulfilling practice.

As you become more attuned to your body, you might discover that external factors like temperature and setting also affect sensitivity. A warm bath or shower beforehand can relax the muscles, making P-Spot stimulation more comfortable. Similarly, an inviting, serene environment can put you at ease. Small elements—soft music, dim lighting, a cozy blanket—can collectively create a space where you feel safe and relaxed enough to explore deeper.

Advanced techniques, such as combining P-Spot stimulation with breathwork or pelvic floor exercises, can further aid in managing sensitivity. These practices increase blood flow and relaxation in the pelvic region, creating a more receptive state. Experimenting with rhythmic breathing or Kegel exercises might seem unrelated at first, but they can significantly enhance your control over sensations, making them more predictable and less overwhelming.

Lastly, remember that sensitivity is not a limitation but an invitation to explore your body's nuanced language. It's about finding a balance between intensity and comfort, between anticipation and fulfillment. Celebrating small victories along the way—whether that's experiencing prolonged pleasure for the first time or simply feeling more at ease with the process—can empower you to continue this intimate journey.

In essence, dealing with sensitivity in P-Spot stimulation requires a blend of patience, communication, and self-awareness. Every person's journey will be unique, shaped by individual thresholds and preferences. Embrace this exploration with gentle curiosity, and you'll find that sensitivity, far from being a barrier, becomes a doorway to deeper, more profound pleasure.

Enhancing Comfort

P-spot stimulation, though incredibly rewarding, can present challenges that make comfort a paramount concern. Achieving comfort can significantly enhance the pleasure derived from P-spot exploration, whether alone or with a partner. The body's readiness plays a crucial role in this process, making it essential to approach stimulation with patience and an understanding of one's own physical and emotional boundaries.

First, let's address the importance of relaxation. Stress or anxiety can lead to muscle tension, particularly in the pelvic area, which can exacerbate discomfort during P-spot stimulation. Deep breathing exercises, progressive muscle relaxation, and even mindfulness practices can be valuable tools in readying the body. Creating a serene environment with dim lighting, relaxing music, or aromatherapy can also contribute to a more relaxed state.

Another cornerstone of comfort is ample lubrication. The rectum does not produce its own lubrication, making the use of an appropriate, high-quality lubricant critical. Silicone-based lubricants are often recommended due to their long-lasting nature and smooth texture. However, it's essential to conduct a patch test first to ensure there are no allergic reactions or sensitivities. Don't hesitate to reapply as needed to maintain a slick surface and minimize friction.

Start slow. Gentle initial stimulation can pave the way for more profound sensations later on. Begin by focusing on external massage around the perineum and anus to increase blood flow and sensitivity. Gradual insertion with gentle, teasing movements can help the body acclimate. The goal is to ease into it, observing how your body reacts and adjusting accordingly.

When it comes to positioning, personal preference reigns supreme, but experimentation can be enlightening. Some find comfort in lying on their back with knees bent, while others may prefer a side-lying position or being on all fours. Comfort can often be enhanced by supporting cushions or pillows to relieve pressure and allow for better relaxation of the pelvic muscles. Trying different angles and positions could uncover new realms of comfort and pleasure.

Acknowledging and managing sensitivity is another crucial aspect. The prostate area can be extremely sensitive, and an overly vigorous approach can lead to discomfort. It's vital to use a tender touch and to communicate openly if exploring with a partner. If engaging solo, tune into your body's signals to gauge pressure and motion that feels right. Sensitivity varies greatly, so what works can often depend on the day and your current physical and emotional state.

Incorporating mindfulness can make a significant difference. Being present in the moment and paying attention to the sensations can deepen the experience. Mindfulness allows you to focus on the pleasurable aspects, easing anxiety and promoting relaxation. Encouraging a mindset of self-compassion and patience can turn any concerns about discomfort into a journey of self-discovery and pleasure.

The role of communication cannot be overstated, especially when involving a partner. Sharing your preferences and boundaries openly fosters a supportive atmosphere. Establishing safe words or signals can be incredibly helpful, ensuring comfort remains a priority throughout the exploration. Mutual respect and understanding can transform an intimate experience into a profound connection.

Using toys specifically designed for P-spot stimulation can also aid in comfort. These toys are ergonomically designed to target the prostate with precision, often featuring curved or angled shapes that facilitate easier access. Vibrations and pulsations can further enhance comfort and pleasure, providing varied sensations without applying too much pressure. Always start with smaller, beginner-friendly toys to build comfort and confidence.

Lastly, taking breaks when needed is crucial. There's no need to power through discomfort. Pausing to regroup and evaluate how you're feeling can prevent any negative associations with P-spot stimulation. Remember, exploring sexual pleasure is a personal journey and there's no right or wrong timeline. Taking your time can ensure that the experience remains positive and fulfilling.

Enhancing comfort in P-spot stimulation is a holistic process that involves physical readiness, mental tranquility, and open communication. This approach not only minimizes discomfort but also enhances the overall pleasure and satisfaction that P-spot stimulation can provide. By prioritizing comfort, you pave the way for a richer and more enjoyable exploration of this deeply intimate and rewarding aspect of sexual pleasure.

Chapter 20:
Myths and Misconceptions
About the G-Spot

The G-Spot, often shrouded in myths and misconceptions, has long fascinated and perplexed many seeking to understand its mysteries. Contrary to popular belief, the G-Spot is not an elusive "magic button" guaranteed to provide instant pleasure, nor is its existence uniformly experienced by everyone. Scientific research suggests that the G-Spot is best understood as a sensitive area within the front vaginal wall, varying significantly in sensitivity and response among individuals. This chapter aims to unravel these myths, shedding light on the diverse experiences of G-Spot stimulation, emphasizing that pleasure is unique to each person. By dispelling these misconceptions, we hope to encourage a more comprehensive and personalized exploration of sexual pleasure, empowering readers with knowledge grounded in both science and real-life experiences.

Popular Beliefs Debunked

When it comes to the G-spot, misconceptions abound, and they often overshadow the more nuanced realities of G-spot stimulation. One popular yet erroneous belief is that the G-spot is a magical button, almost like a sexual switch that, when pressed, guarantees an instant and explosive orgasm. This oversimplification not only sets unrealistic expectations but also can lead to frustration and disappointment for individuals or couples exploring this area.

The truth is far more intricate and fascinating. The G-spot, named after Dr. Ernst Gräfenberg, is not a single spot but a sensitive area within the anterior vaginal wall. Its responsiveness can vary significantly from person to person. Some may find that their G-spot responds dramatically, while others may not feel much. This variability is perfectly normal and highlights the importance of exploration and open-mindedness in sexual experiences.

Another entrenched myth is that all women possess a G-spot and that its stimulation is essential for sexual fulfillment. While scientific studies indicate that many women do have an area of heightened sensitivity that could be described as the G-spot, not everyone might experience it in the same way. Moreover, sexual pleasure is multifaceted and doesn't hinge on the G-spot alone. The journey to discovering one's unique pleasure points is an individual experience, resonating differently for each person.

Society often posits that G-spot stimulation must lead to ejaculation, sometimes referred to as "female ejaculation" or "squirting." This is also a misconception drenched in hyperbole and misinformation. Not every woman will experience ejaculation through G-spot stimulation, and for those who do, the experience and volume can vary widely. Ejaculation, like orgasm, should not be considered the ultimate goal but rather one of the many expressions of sexual pleasure. Placing unwarranted emphasis on it can detract from the broader and more essential facets of intimate connection and mutual satisfaction.

We also encounter the belief that G-spot orgasms are somehow superior to other types of orgasms, such as clitoral orgasms. This hierarchy of pleasure is misleading and simplistic. The idea that one type of orgasm is "better" than another feeds into a competitive and goal-oriented mindset about sex. In reality, every individual's sexual response is unique, and clitoral, G-spot, and blended orgasms can all provide distinct but equally valuable and enriching experiences.

Many people also mistakenly believe that locating and stimulating the G-spot requires complex techniques or specialized knowledge, which can intimidate those new to the concept. While some techniques may be more effective for certain individuals, the most crucial elements are often open communication and intuitive exploration. A sense of curiosity and patience often leads to greater discoveries than any prescriptive methods found in a how-to guide. Comfort and relaxation are key, and the journey of finding pleasure should be just as enjoyable as the destination.

The myth that G-spot stimulation is only pleasurable when performed in a specific way or certain positions is equally unfounded. In truth, the best techniques and positions for G-spot stimulation vary dramatically among individuals and couples. What works well for one person might not be as effective for another. This is why flexibility and experimentation are vital components of sexual exploration. Trying different angles, motions, and levels of pressure can help in discovering what feels best for each unique body.

Another prevailing myth is that G-spot stimulation is only for younger women, neglecting the fact that sexual pleasure evolves over a lifetime. Age doesn't diminish the G-spot's capacity for responsiveness. Instead, life experience and a deeper understanding of one's body often enhance the richness of sexual encounters. Both individuals and couples can continue to explore and appreciate the nuances of G-spot pleasure at any age, finding joy and connection through various stages of life.

There's also confusion stemming from the blend of myths around anatomy and physiological responses. One widespread trope is that G-spot stimulation is purely a physical act, disregarding the psychological and emotional components of sexual pleasure. In reality, the mind-body connection plays a critical role in how we experience sexual sensations. Indeed, the anticipation, emotional intimacy, and psychological readiness often enhance physical stimulation and amplify the overall experience.

It's also important to debunk the misconception that achieving G-spot pleasure requires a partner with a specific genital size. This belief not only excludes and alienates certain individuals but also misunderstands the essence of intimate exploration. The size of a partner's genitalia is far less important than the techniques used, the attentiveness shown, and the mutual understanding developed between partners. Small, focused efforts often yield greater satisfaction than attempts to conform to size-based myths.

When tackling these myths, one must also address the gendered stereotypes attached to the G-spot. For example, the notion that a woman's pleasure is less complex or less important than a man's can seep into understandings of G-spot stimulation. Emphasizing mutual pleasure and egalitarian approaches to exploring each other's bodies enhances the emotional and physical satisfaction for all involved. Dispelling these myths helps create a more inclusive narrative around sexual pleasure.

In light of these debunked myths, what stands out most is the need for comprehensive sex education and open dialogue surrounding sexual pleasure. By encouraging a culture of learning and genuine curiosity, we can navigate beyond the myths and embrace a more fulfilling and realistic view of sexual intimacy. Conversations that focus on actual experiences, scientific understanding, and emotional connections pave the way for more enriching explorations of the G-spot and beyond.

The complexities of sexual relationships and pleasure cannot be gleaned through myths or misconceptions. Only through honest inquiry, mutual respect, and a willingness to dismantle old beliefs can we truly appreciate the wonders of the G-spot. Empowering individuals and couples to explore their bodies and communicate openly about their needs not only debunks these popular beliefs but also fosters deeper connection and joy in their intimate lives.

As we shed light on these myths, it's essential to remember that the G-spot is just one element within the grand tapestry of human sexuality. Celebrating diverse pathways to pleasure reaffirms the idea that there is no one-size-fits-all approach to sexual fulfillment. Exploring with openness and without judgment fosters a healthier, more satisfying sexual experience for everyone. Each step taken away from myth and towards understanding is a step towards a more empowered and enlightened sexual existence.

The Reality of G-Spot Pleasure

Delving into the reality of G-Spot pleasure requires us to strip away the myths and misconceptions that have clouded its true nature. For many, the G-Spot is shrouded in mystery, with some doubting its very existence. Let's be clear: the G-Spot is a real part of the female anatomy. It is not an elusive legend. However, understanding its complexities and the pleasures it can provide involves more than just locating it physically.

First, it's essential to recognize that the G-Spot is not a standalone entity but an extension of the broader clitoral network. This erogenous zone, nestled on the anterior wall of the vagina, about a third of the way in, comprises a dense bundle of nerve endings, glands, and spongy tissue. When stimulated, it can engorge and become aroused, leading to heightened sensations and, for many, profound pleasure. But the pathway to this pleasure is not uniform for every individual.

Expecting a universal reaction to G-Spot stimulation does a disservice to oneself and one's partner. The journey to discovering G-Spot pleasure is deeply personal. For some, the touch of a fingertip or a specifically designed toy ignites instant, electrifying responses. For others, it may require a more nuanced approach, incorporating arousal from other sources like the clitoris. These variations are not anomalies but rather reflections of the diverse landscape of human sexual pleasure.

An often-overlooked aspect of G-Spot pleasure is its context within the overall sexual experience. Emotional connection, mental arousal, and physical relaxation play critical roles. Anxiety or stress can blunt sensitivity, while a romantic setting or intimate foreplay can amplify sensations. The G-Spot thrives in an environment where all forms of arousal—mental, emotional, and physical—intersect.

Perhaps a more elusive, yet impactful, component of G-Spot pleasure is the potential for G-Spot orgasms. These can differ significantly from clitoral orgasms in intensity and sensation. While clitoral orgasms often build up quickly and result in rapid, concentrated bursts of pleasure, G-Spot orgasms can involve a deeper, more profound release. Some describe them as waves of pleasure that flow through the entire body, more sustained and involving different muscle groups, including the pelvic floor.

Given this complexity, it's crucial to approach G-Spot exploration with patience and openness. Instead of a checklist of techniques or positions, think of it as an ongoing conversation with your body. Communication with your partner, if you're not exploring solo, also can't be overstated. Verbal and non-verbal feedback can be integral to tuning into the unique responses of the G-Spot.

Furthermore, the G-Spot's pleasures aren't just about the sexual act itself; they reflect a journey of self-discovery and connection. The process of locating and enjoying G-Spot stimulation can foster deeper intimacy and trust between partners. It encourages a level of vulnerability and openness that can be profoundly enriching to a relationship. Knowing that your partner is attuned to your body's responses, and that you are exploring this pleasure together, can build an unspoken bond that transcends the physical.

The tools of the trade also play a significant role in enhancing G-Spot pleasure. While manual stimulation with fingers remains a classic approach, the modern market offers a variety of specialized toys designed to provide targeted G-Spot stimulation. These include curved dildos, vibrating devices, and dual-action toys that also engage the clitoris. The effectiveness of these tools can vary, and what works wonders for one individual might not do as much for another. This underscores the importance of experimentation and personalization in sexual exploration.

It's also worth mentioning that the G-Spot can play a role in experiences beyond the physical sensation—particularly, the phenomenon of female ejaculation. While it is not universally experienced, some women report ejaculation coinciding with G-Spot stimulation. This can add another layer of intensity to G-Spot pleasure, although it's not a universal marker of success or the ultimate goal.

Finally, we must look at the broader cultural understanding of G-Spot pleasure. Historically, there has been a tendency to either overhype or downplay its importance. This binary thinking has contributed to feelings of inadequacy or frustration when personal experiences don't align with exaggerated claims or skepticism. By embracing a nuanced, informed perspective, we can normalize diverse experiences and ultimately foster a healthier, more holistic view of sexual pleasure.

In essence, the reality of G-Spot pleasure is multifaceted and deeply personal. It requires an openness to explore and a willingness to understand one's body in new ways. It's a journey that can lead to greater sexual fulfillment and deeper emotional connections, both with oneself and with a partner. Breaking free from myths and approaching G-Spot pleasure with curiosity and empathy can transform not just your sexual experiences, but also your relationship with your own body and sexuality.

Chapter 21:
Myths and Misconceptions
About the P-Spot

Myths and misconceptions about the P-spot have long clouded an area ripe with potential for profound pleasure. For many, the term "P-spot" conjures images that are as confusing as they are inaccurate. One of the most pervasive myths is that exploring the P-spot is inherently uncomfortable or even painful, but this couldn't be further from the truth. With proper understanding and technique, P-spot stimulation can be an incredibly rewarding part of intimate experiences. Another common misconception is that this form of stimulation is reserved solely for a particular gender or orientation, but it is essential to recognize that pleasure knows no bounds and is a universal aspect of human experience. By dispelling these myths, we can break down the barriers that prevent individuals from exploring this aspect of their sexuality and instead embrace it with curiosity and confidence.

Challenging Common Beliefs

When it comes to sexual pleasure and anatomy, the P-Spot, or prostate, often remains shrouded in mystery and misconceptions. Much like the G-Spot for women, the P-Spot's role in male sexual health is frequently misunderstood. At the heart of these misconceptions lies a complex web of societal norms, inadequate sex education, and sometimes, the challenge of communicating openly about such intimate matters.

One common belief is that exploring the P-Spot is solely about achieving intense orgasms. While prostate stimulation can indeed lead to profound sexual pleasure, limiting the discussion to orgasms alone oversimplifies its significance. The prostate is a crucial part of male anatomy with important health benefits; its stimulation can lead not only to heightened sexual experiences but also serve as a preventative practice against certain prostate-related ailments. Thus, reframing the conversation can allow for a broader understanding of the P-Spot's multifaceted role in male health.

Historically, the P-Spot has sometimes been inaccurately categorized as being solely of interest to individuals identifying as homosexual. This belief is not just unfounded but also harmful, as it perpetuates stigma and discourages many men from exploring a potentially enriching aspect of their sexuality. The reality is that prostate pleasure knows no boundaries around sexual orientation. Acknowledging this can foster a more inclusive and enriching dialogue that benefits all men, regardless of their sexual identity.

Let's also tackle the misconception that P-Spot stimulation is inherently uncomfortable or painful. This belief sometimes arises from initial attempts that may have lacked proper technique or sufficient preparation. Just as any other form of sexual exploration, prostate stimulation requires a balance of patience, the right technique, and open communication with one's partner or oneself. Using adequate lubrication, adopting comfortable positions, and moving at a pace that's right for the individual are essential factors in turning any discomfort into an experience of heightened pleasure.

Another myth worth debunking is the idea that P-Spot stimulation is unsanitary. Proper hygiene practices can mitigate most concerns related to cleanliness. Just as with any other intimate act, a bit of preparation goes a long way in ensuring both partners feel secure and comfortable. Washing hands and toys before and after use, as well as ensuring the anal area is clean, can create an environment where the focus remains on pleasure and intimacy.

There's also the notion that discussing or exploring the P-Spot disrupts masculinity or makes it seem fragile. This belief is deeply rooted in cultural norms that unfairly equate masculinity with dominance and invulnerability. Shifting away from these restrictive paradigms towards a healthier, more holistic approach to male sexuality can be liberating. Embracing prostate stimulation as a normal, satisfying part of sexual exploration can foster deeper self-awareness and even improve overall intimate relationships.

Additionally, some men worry that focusing on the P-Spot will detract from traditional forms of sexual pleasure, such as penile stimulation. In reality, many find that incorporating prostate play can significantly enhance their sexual experiences. Combining penile and prostate stimulation, for instance, can create a synergistic effect, leading to orgasms that are often described as more intense and fulfilling than through penile stimulation alone.

The stigma associated with prostate stimulation can also lead to unspoken fears of judgment or ridicule. It is vital to establish a culture of openness and mutual respect in intimate relationships. Honesty about desires and boundaries can foster a stronger connection and trust between partners. Education and open dialogue can combat the stigma and create a more accepting environment where both partners feel free to explore and express their desires without fear of judgment.

Medical myths also contribute to the reluctance to explore the P-Spot. Some men worry that stimulating the prostate could cause medical issues. In truth, regular prostate massage has been shown to improve prostate health, potentially lowering the risk of prostatitis and other related conditions. Prostate stimulation, when done correctly and safely, is beneficial rather than harmful.

Lastly, there's the belief that only certain individuals, perhaps those who are "adventurous" or "kinky," would enjoy or benefit from P-Spot stimulation. This stereotype does a disservice to many who might enjoy prostate play but feel it's beyond the scope of "normal" sexual behavior. Recognizing that sexual pleasure and exploration are deeply personal and unique to each individual can help dismantle these restrictive notions. Everyone deserves to explore what brings them pleasure in a safe and consensual manner.

Breaking down these misconceptions is essential for men to fully embrace their sexual health and pleasure. Understanding the P-Spot and its benefits can lead to a more holistic approach towards male sexuality, enhancing both solo and partnered experiences. The journey towards sexual pleasure and health is personal and ever-evolving. Dispelling myths allows men to step into a world of deeper self-discovery and pleasure, unbounded by harmful misconceptions or societal judgments.

Factual Information

When discussing the P-Spot, it's crucial to dispel myths with cold, hard facts. The P-Spot, another name for the prostate gland in individuals assigned male at birth, is often misunderstood and surrounded by misconceptions. This section aims to provide clear, factual information to guide you in your exploration.

The prostate is a small gland located just below the bladder and in front of the rectum. It is part of the male reproductive system and plays a vital role in sexual function. The gland is typically the size of a walnut and surrounds the urethra, which is the tube that carries urine and semen out of the body.

Although the P-Spot or prostate is often cited as a pleasure center for men, it's essential to understand that the sensation derived from P-Spot stimulation can vary significantly from person to person. For some, it can lead to intense pleasure and even result in powerful orgasms, often described as different from penile stimulation orgasms. However, others may not find the same level of pleasure or may experience discomfort or pain, especially if they have underlying medical conditions such as prostatitis or prostate cancer.

Several studies have shown that the prostate is highly sensitive due to the presence of numerous nerve endings. This neural richness is what potentially makes prostate stimulation pleasurable for many. It's an area that can be explored to heighten one's overall sexual experience, but it requires an informed and gentle approach.

Moreover, the history of the prostate being recognized as a pleasure point varies across cultures and medical practices. While some societies and medical literature have long acknowledged the sexual potential of the prostate, it is only in more recent years that Western cultures have more openly discussed and explored the pleasures of P-Spot stimulation without stigma.

Another important fact is related to safety and proper technique when exploring P-Spot stimulation. For novices and even experienced individuals, there's always a risk of injuring the delicate tissues surrounding the prostate if one isn't careful. This emphasizes the need to use lubricants generously and proceed with patience, avoiding rushed or overly forceful methods. Hygiene, too, cannot be overstressed since the area around the P-Spot is prone to infections if not properly cleaned.

Despite the factual underpinnings, numerous myths aim to deter men from exploring their P-Spot, often couched in baseless fears about sexuality and masculinity. One of the most pervasive myths is the unfounded belief that enjoying P-Spot stimulation is linked to one's sexual orientation. The truth is that P-Spot pleasure has nothing to do with orientation; it is purely about understanding and maximizing one's body's potential for pleasure.

Additionally, there's a misconception that stimulating the P-Spot requires professional medical assistance or invasive procedures, which is far from the truth. With proper guidance and care, P-Spot exploration can be comfortably and effectively conducted in the privacy of one's own home. Learning about the P-Spot should empower individuals and couples to enrich their sexual experiences, dismissing the myths that surround this misunderstood topic.

In essence, the P-Spot stands as an important aspect of male sexual health and pleasure. The factual information above aims to equip you with the necessary knowledge to explore and appreciate the P-Spot intelligently and safely. It's about embracing a holistic approach—acknowledging anatomy, dismissing myths, and prioritizing personal comfort and pleasure preferences. With these insights, you'll be well on your way to understanding and potentially integrating P-Spot play into your intimate life, should you choose to explore it.

Chapter 22:
Advanced Techniques for
G-Spot Stimulation

The journey into advanced G-Spot stimulation begins with an understanding that each individual's body is unique, requiring a personalized approach to uncover deeper sensations. Elevate your intimate experiences by experimenting with various pressures, rhythms, and angles to discover what specific combination unlocks unparalleled pleasure. Use the "come hither" motion with your fingers or try different toys designed for precision targeting. Communicate openly and tenderly with your partner, fostering an environment where safety and trust flourish, thus enhancing both emotional and physical connection. With practice, you'll build an intuitive skillset that transforms each encounter into a symphony of bliss. This chapter will empower you to explore and harness these techniques, allowing you to transcend ordinary experiences and achieve extraordinary intimacy.

Exploring Deeper Sensations

Delving into the realm of deeper sensations when it comes to G-Spot stimulation is like opening a new chapter in a book you thought you had already read. It's simultaneously familiar and entirely novel, beckoning you to explore its depths with curiosity and eagerness. This journey isn't just about physical techniques but also involves psychological readiness and emotional connection.

When aiming to reach deeper sensations, the key is to go beyond the superficial layers of touch. It's about tapping into the nuanced responses that your body can offer. The G-Spot, an area already known for its sensitivity, becomes an even more potent source of pleasure when you understand how to engage it deeply. This involves more than pressure; it's about rhythm, angle, and the context of the stimuli.

The foundation of deeper sensations lies in mastering gradual and intentional buildup. One effective technique involves a rhythmic 'come hither' motion with a finger, knuckle, or toy designed specifically for G-Spot stimulation. This motion, consistent yet adaptable, gradually awakens the deeper layers of the G-Spot and invites prolonged, rolling waves of pleasure.

To further explore these deeper sensations, consider varying the pressure and speed in response to your body's feedback. It's like learning a dance where each movement is responsive and considerate of your partner—a perfect balance between leading and being led.

Advanced techniques also often include the interplay of temperature and texture. Using warmed or chilled toys can add a thrilling new dimension to the experience. Likewise, toys with varied textures—ridges, bumps, or curves—can stimulate different parts of the G-Spot in unique ways. Experimenting with these elements can unlock new realms of sensation that were previously dormant.

You might find that deeper G-Spot stimulation can evoke mixed emotions—intense pleasure, profound satisfaction, and even emotional release. This is a natural response, one that speaks to the deep connection between physical and psychological experiences. Allow yourself to fully experience these emotions without judgment; they are an integral part of your journey.

Another important aspect of exploring deeper sensations is understanding the role of consistent practice and patience. Developing the refined sensitivity required for deeper G-Spot stimulation isn't an overnight process. It involves repeated exploration, an openness to learning, and a willingness to listen to your body's nuanced signals.

Meanwhile, communicating openly with a partner becomes essential in partnered play. Relay your needs, desires, and responses clearly. This not only enhances the physical aspect of G-Spot stimulation but also fortifies the emotional intimacy between both partners. Trust and vulnerability become the fertile ground from which deeper sensations can flourish.

Transitioning from one state of arousal to another with intention helps in accessing deeper sensations. Instead of focusing solely on the destination of orgasm, immerse yourself in the journey. Savor each wave of pleasure as it builds, and allow each moment to be fully experienced.

Complementing G-Spot stimulation with other forms of arousal, such as clitoral or nipple stimulation, can also amplify the depth of sensation. Combining these different pleasure sources can lead to a more immersive and integrative experience. It's an approach that embraces the holistic nature of human sexual response.

For many, the journey toward exploring deeper sensations may also include breathwork and mindful awareness. Practicing deep, rhythmic breathing can enhance oxygen flow and relaxation, creating a conducive environment for receiving deeper pleasure. Being mentally present, without distractions, allows for a fuller, more profound experience.

Finally, set the stage with an ambiance that promotes relaxation and intimacy. Soft lighting, calming music, and a serene, comfortable environment prepare your mind and body for a deeper connection. This attention to setting isn't mere aesthetic; it's part of the sensory tapestry that enhances the overall experience.

Exploring deeper sensations with the G-Spot opens up a world of possibilities, where physical pleasure meets emotional richness and psychological fulfillment. It's a journey best undertaken with patience, intentionality, and an open heart. Whether solo or with a partner, this advanced exploration offers a path to profound self-awareness and intimate connection, enriching your sexual landscape in ways that are as unique as they are powerful.

Enhancing Skillsets

Developing advanced techniques for G-Spot stimulation isn't just about mechanics and methodology; it's about honing your sensibilities and deepening your connection with both your body and your partner. Mastery comes from a blend of knowledge, practice, and intuition. As you journey through the realms of intimate exploration, enhancing your skillset becomes a continuous, evolving process.

Start by cultivating a deeper awareness of your own or your partner's physiological responses. This means paying close attention to subtle cues such as changes in breathing, skin flushes, and muscle contractions. These signals can guide you in fine-tuning your techniques, understanding what feels good and what doesn't, and adjusting your approach accordingly. Building this sensory acuity takes time and practice, but it forms the foundation of truly advanced G-Spot stimulation.

Interactive learning is another key component. Engage in open dialogue with your partner about what feels pleasurable and what sensations are most intense. Encourage honest feedback, as this will enable both of you to refine your techniques and discover new pathways to pleasure. Remember, the journey of enhancing your skillset is mutual, involving constant communication and shared exploration.

Exploring different angles and pressures is essential in mastering G-Spot stimulation. The G-Spot isn't a static point but a dynamic area that can respond differently to varied touches. Gentle caresses with gradual increases in pressure can awaken and stimulate the sensitive tissues effectively. Experimentation is crucial: sometimes a slow, deliberate motion could elicit stronger responses than rapid, repetitive actions. Find what resonates by varying both your speed and technique.

The rhythm you set is another aspect where skill development plays a role. Syncing your movements with the natural ebb and flow of arousal can create a more immersive and fulfilling experience. Pay attention to the tempo of breathing and the rhythm of muscle contractions. Matching your movements to these natural rhythms can amplify sensations and lead to more profound pleasure.

Another powerful technique to enhance G-Spot stimulation involves integrating other erogenous zones into your practice. Combining G-Spot with clitoral stimulation can significantly heighten arousal and lead to more intense orgasms. Use one hand or a toy to stimulate the clitoris while the other focuses on the G-Spot. This dual stimulation can create a symphony of sensations, overwhelming and delighting the senses.

For a more dynamic approach, consider incorporating different positions that facilitate better access to the G-Spot. Positions such as the classic missionary with a pillow under the hips or the woman-on-top gives more control over the angle and depth of penetration. These positions allow for varied pressure and rhythm, making discovering what works best for you or your partner easier.

Toys designed for G-Spot stimulation can also elevate your skillset. Many toys are specifically crafted to target the G-Spot with precise angles and textures. Experiment with different shapes and sizes to find the perfect match. Vibrating G-Spot toys can add an extra layer of stimulation, providing consistent pressure and vibrations that manual techniques might not achieve.

As you advance your techniques, it's important to remain attuned to the emotional and psychological aspects of G-Spot stimulation. Emotional connectivity enhances physical experiences. Creating a safe, intimate, and trusting environment will facilitate relaxation and openness. Practices such as deep breathing, mindfulness, and mutual reassurance can help in building this emotional connection, making the physical sensations even more satisfying.

Personal practice and exploration are equally important. Masturbation isn't just about pleasure; it's an opportunity to explore your body's responses. Discovering what movements and pressures feel best provides a roadmap for partnered play. Don't shy away from experimenting with new techniques or tools during solo sessions. This empowers you with knowledge and confidence, which you can then bring into partnered encounters.

Training your muscles through Kegel exercises can also enhance your G-Spot skillset. Strengthening the pelvic floor muscles increases control and sensation, allowing for more intense contractions during orgasm. Practice contractions during play; this can enhance the G-Spot experience for both you and your partner.

While honing technical skills is vital, remember that the ultimate goal of enhancing your G-Spot stimulation skillset is to foster a deeper sense of connection and mutual pleasure. Approach each encounter with a spirit of curiosity and openness. Embrace each sensation, each feedback, and each moment as a step towards mastering the art of intimate exploration.

Reflecting on your experiences and discussing them with your partner can also enhance your skillset. Post-play conversations can reveal insights that may not be apparent during the heat of the moment. Talk about what worked, what didn't, and what you'd like to try next time. This reflective practice can deepen your understanding and improve your techniques over time.

Never underestimate the power of continuous learning. Stay informed about the latest research, tips, and advancements in sexual health and pleasure. Attend workshops, read books, and engage with communities that focus on sexual wellness. This ongoing quest for knowledge ensures that your approach remains fresh, innovative, and satisfying.

Remember, enhancing your G-Spot skillset is a journey, not a destination. Celebrate the milestones, however small, and cherish the growth you experience along the way. Each step you take towards improving your techniques enriches your intimate life, bringing you closer to a fulfilling and joyous sexual connection.

In conclusion, improving your skillset for G-Spot stimulation is a multifaceted endeavor that blends physiologic understanding, technical skills, emotional intelligence, and continuous learning. Embrace the process with enthusiasm and an open heart, and you'll find your intimate experiences deepening and flourishing in ways you never imagined.

Chapter 23:
Advanced Techniques for
P-Spot Stimulation

Building upon foundational knowledge of P-Spot stimulation, this chapter delves into techniques designed for those ready to elevate their experiences. It begins with a focus on refining touch and pressure, essential for heightening sensation and achieving deeper satisfaction. Emphasizing the importance of communication, it explores the synchronization between partners, allowing for an intimate and responsive exchange. For solo adventurers, advanced breathing exercises are introduced to enhance relaxation and intensify pleasure. Special attention is given to exploring various positions and the use of specialized toys, each providing unique angles and pressures to maximize P-Spot engagement. The chapter encourages embracing vulnerability and trust, pivotal in deepening the emotional and physical connection, ultimately transforming the experience from mere stimulation to an enriching journey of mutual discovery and bliss.

Techniques for Experienced Individuals

Delving into advanced techniques for P-spot stimulation is akin to a sculptor refining their masterpiece over time. It requires a nuanced understanding of one's own body or one's partner's, wrapped in a deep sense of trust and adventurism. As you embark on mastering these advanced methods, keep in mind that the journey itself is a significant part of the experience.

One of the foremost techniques for experienced individuals involves leveraging rhythmic contractions. These contractions, also known as kegels, engage the pelvic floor muscles, which can intensify the sensations experienced during P-spot stimulation. Practicing consistent and deliberate kegels can help in building muscle control, thereby allowing for more controlled and heightened arousal. The beauty of this technique lies in its simplicity and the profound impact it can have on sexual satisfaction.

Exploring different angles and positions can significantly enhance pleasure. While the basic techniques might focus on the simplest, most direct routes, venturing into more varied positions can bring about different sensations and deeper stimulation. Some positions might foster a more intimate bond with a partner, while others can unlock new realms of personal pleasure. Experimentation is key, and what works better for one person may not hold the same enchantment for another.

Toys designed for P-spot stimulation open up a world of possibilities for those willing to explore. Advanced users might find that incorporating vibrators or other prostate massagers can considerably enhance the experience. These devices often come with different settings and features, allowing users to customize their experience. The vibrations can provide consistent pressure on the P-spot, leading to more powerful orgasms. It's important to spend time getting familiar with the device, starting with lower settings and gradually increasing intensity to find what feels best.

Synchronization of breath with stimulation can also magnify the experience. Breathwork is a powerful tool that can amplify sensory input and help individuals remain in an aroused state for longer periods. Inhaling deeply and exhaling slowly, in sync with the rhythm of stimulation, can lead to a more immersive and connected experience. Additionally, breath control can assist in tempering the intensity of sensations, thus extending the duration of pleasure.

Communication remains a cornerstone even (or especially) in advanced practices. If P-spot stimulation is a shared endeavor with a partner, discussing boundaries, preferences, and experiences openly can prevent misunderstandings and enhance mutual satisfaction. The emotional intimacy engendered through such open dialogues can elevate the physical experience, creating a richer, more fulfilling connection.

Understanding one's arousal arc adds another layer to P-spot mastery. The arousal arc describes the journey from initial arousal to climax and includes understanding one's peak moments and how to prolong and intensify these sensations. Experienced individuals often play with edging techniques, which involve nearing climax and then backing off to heighten anticipation. This can make the actual orgasm more powerful and satisfying.

A nuanced understanding of lubrication can't be overstressed. Experienced individuals often find that certain lubricants work better for specific types of stimulation. Silicone-based lubricants, for instance, might offer a smoother, longer-lasting glide, which can be particularly useful during extended play sessions. On the other hand, water-based lubricants might be favorable for their ease of cleanup even if they require more frequent application.

Initiating mindfulness practices can bring a new depth to P-spot play. Being present in the moment, focusing on the sensations and emotions as they arise, can make the experience more fulfilling. Mindfulness helps in cultivating a sense of connection with oneself or with a partner, enriching the overall sexual experience. This practice can also aid in identifying what specifically enhances or detracts from pleasure, allowing for more personalized and satisfying encounters.

For those who incorporate P-spot stimulation into their regular sexual repertoire, blending it with other forms of stimulation can lead to unique and extraordinary experiences. For instance, combining anal and penile stimulation can create an interplay of sensations that amplify overall pleasure. This dual stimulation can be particularly gratifying when the timing and rhythm are synchronized, elevating the sexual experience to new heights.

Moreover, tuning into the subtleties of emotional responses can deepen your connection to P-spot stimulation. Emotional factors—such as trust, love, and intimacy—can significantly influence the physical sensations experienced. Recognizing and embracing these emotional responses doesn't only heighten the physical pleasure but also enriches the overall intimacy between partners.

In advanced explorations, pay heed to the body's reaction to different stimuli and adjust accordingly. The body's responsiveness can change from one session to another, making adaptability a crucial skill. It could be the shift in pressure, the introduction of a new angle, or even a change in rhythm that brings about a new dimension of pleasure.

Another advanced technique involves the use of external aids like hot or cold temperatures. Introducing temperature play can excite the nerve endings and bring about unique and intense sensations. A cool metal toy or a warm, lubricated hand can drastically change the sensory experience, adding an element of surprise and novelty.

Finally, cultivating a ritual of aftercare is just as crucial as the stimulation itself. Aftercare involves activities that help relax and comfort individuals after intense sexual experiences. This could be a warm bath, gentle caresses, or simply lying together and talking about the experience. Aftercare helps in grounding oneself after intense sensations and emotional intimacy, further solidifying the bond between partners or deepening one's own self-awareness.

Advanced P-spot stimulation isn't just about achieving more profound orgasms; it's about forging a deeper connection with oneself or one's partner. The skills and techniques involved require practice, patience, and a willingness to explore and communicate. By embracing these elements, one can truly unlock the full potential of P-spot pleasure.

Deepening the Experience

As you become more experienced with P-Spot stimulation, you may find yourself seeking ways to enhance and deepen the sensations. There's something profoundly rewarding about taking a well-known technique and evolving it into a more intimate and profound experience. This chapter aims to explore advanced methods and approaches to P-Spot stimulation that are designed to elevate your pleasure and emotional connection, both in solo play and with a partner.

Firstly, it is essential to acknowledge that deepening the experience is not solely about physical techniques. The mind plays a significant role in sexual pleasure, and fostering a positive and open mindset can dramatically transform your encounters. Emotional readiness and mental relaxation are crucial; try practicing mindfulness or meditative techniques before beginning P-Spot play. This can help ground you in the present moment, making each touch and sensation more vivid and impactful.

For those who are already comfortable with basic techniques, advanced approaches may include experimenting with different types of pressure and rhythm. In contrast to lighter, rhythmic strokes, applying firm, sustained pressure to the P-Spot can yield a profound sense of fullness and intense pleasure. Use your finger or a well-designed toy to explore different angles and depths, paying close attention to how each variation affects your sensations. Variety in tempo can also yield surprising results; this might mean slowing down and savoring each movement, or incorporating sudden, unexpected changes in rhythm to keep the experience dynamic and exciting.

Breathwork is another powerful tool in deepening your P-Spot experiences. Coordinating your breaths with your movements can create a harmonious flow that amplifies pleasure. Try inhaling deeply and exhaling slowly as you apply pressure or movement to the P-Spot. This synchronization can enhance the body's natural response, making the sensations more intense. Breath also plays a key role in relaxation, reducing any tension that might inhibit pleasure.

Partnered P-Spot stimulation offers a unique opportunity to deepen intimacy and trust between partners. Clear and honest communication is indispensable, creating an environment where both partners feel safe and connected. Discuss boundaries, preferences, and desires openly to ensure a mutually gratifying experience. Utilize eye contact, gentle touch, and verbal affirmations to reinforce emotional intimacy.

One advanced technique is to incorporate simultaneous stimuli, such as combining P-Spot stimulation with other erogenous zones. For instance, integrating penile or scrotal massage while engaging the P-Spot can create a symphony of sensations, enhancing the overall experience. Couples may also experiment with different positions to find what is most comfortable and pleasurable. Positions such as the spooning position or lying on your back with legs elevated can provide optimal angles for reaching the P-Spot.

Toys that are designed specifically for P-Spot stimulation can elevate the experience. These toys often feature ergonomic designs that target the P-Spot with precision. Some advanced toys offer vibrating or pulsating functions, which can add layers of sensation and enhance your experience. Experiment with different shapes, sizes, and settings to find what resonates most with your body.

Another mode of deepening the experience is through edging, which involves bringing yourself or your partner to the brink of orgasm and then stopping before climax. This technique can increase sensitivity and intensify the eventual orgasm, making it more powerful and satisfying. Edging requires patience and self-control but can be incredibly rewarding when done properly.

Exploring advanced lubrication options is another avenue to enhance the P-Spot experience. Some lubricants are designed with warming or cooling agents that can add unique sensations. Additionally, trying out hybrid or silicone-based lubricants might provide a smoother, longer-lasting glide that can make extended sessions more comfortable and pleasurable.

For those more spiritually inclined, integrating elements such as Tantric or Taoist sexual practices can offer a profound depth to P-Spot stimulation. These ancient practices often focus on the harmony between mind, body, and spirit, incorporating breathing exercises, meditation, and specific techniques aimed at channeling sexual energy throughout the body. Such practices can transform a physical act into a deeply spiritual experience.

Finally, consider keeping a journal of your experiences. Documenting what techniques you tried, what worked, and what didn't can provide valuable insights over time. It allows you to track your progress, recognize patterns, and better understand your body's responses. Additionally, sharing this journal with a trusted partner can foster deeper communication and collaborative exploration.

Deepening the experience of P-Spot stimulation is a multifaceted journey that intertwines physical techniques with emotional and mental preparedness. By integrating these advanced strategies, you can elevate your intimate encounters to new heights, fostering a richer, more fulfilling connection with yourself and, if applicable, your partner. The realm of pleasure is boundless, and the only limits are those we set upon ourselves. Embrace the journey and allow yourself the freedom to explore, discover, and enjoy the pleasures that await.

Chapter 24:
Integrating G-Spot Stimulation
into a Healthy Sex Life

To weave G-Spot stimulation into a fulfilling sex life, it's essential to recognize the balance between physical pleasure and emotional intimacy. Begin with open communication with your partner about desires, boundaries, and expectations. This dialogue fosters trust, making exploration more comfortable and mutually rewarding. By combining holistic approaches such as mindfulness and body awareness, you align both mind and body, enhancing the sensations derived from G-Spot stimulation. Remember, the journey is just as important as the destination. Embrace the opportunity to deepen your connection, promote mutual satisfaction, and enrich your overall sexual well-being. Ultimately, integrating these practices into your routine can lead to a healthier and more gratifying intimate life.

Balancing Pleasure and Intimacy

When it comes to integrating G-Spot stimulation into a healthy sex life, the delicate blend of pleasure and intimacy plays a pivotal role. Intimacy, in its purest form, is the emotional closeness shared between partners. It's about feeling connected, loved, and understood beyond the physical sensations. Balancing pleasure and intimacy means acknowledging that while techniques and physical stimulation can amplify sexual pleasure, the true essence of an enriching sex life lies in the harmony between the body and the heart.

Establishing this balance requires open communication. Partners must feel comfortable discussing their desires, boundaries, and any apprehensions that might arise. This conversation doesn't need to be clinical; think of it as an intimate dialogue where both partners express themselves freely. By sharing fantasies, exploring each other's turn-ons, and understanding each other's fears or hesitations, couples lay a foundation for deeper, more meaningful sexual experiences.

Consider the broader context of your relationship. How do you and your partner show affection outside the bedroom? Simple gestures like holding hands, a lingering kiss, or even a loving text message can enhance feelings of intimacy. When sexual encounters are framed within this ongoing emotional connection, the pleasure derived from G-Spot stimulation becomes intertwined with a sense of unity and love.

At times, the euphoria of discovering new heights of pleasure through G-Spot stimulation might lead to focusing primarily on the physical aspects. It's easy to get caught up in mastering techniques or seeking out the next thrilling sensation. But without the underpinning of intimacy, these experiences can feel hollow. Imagine the G-Spot as a gatekeeper to a deeper emotional connection. The key is not just in knowing how to stimulate it but in doing so while maintaining eye contact, sharing tender words, and engaging in mutual exploration.

Some couples find it beneficial to set aside dedicated time for both pleasure-focused sessions and intimacy-building activities. This might look like spending an evening trying out new techniques and another evening simply holding each other, talking, or sharing a bath. By diversifying their intimate interactions, couples can ensure that their sex life is not merely about peak moments of pleasure but also about a continuous journey of connection.

The psychological element cannot be overstated. Deep psychological and emotional bonds can elevate physical pleasure.

When partners feel truly seen and valued, their ability to relax and surrender to sensation increases. Imagine a scenario where both partners are fully attuned to each other's rhythms, desires, and vulnerabilities. The G-Spot becomes not just a physical spot but a touchstone for shared joy and love.

Incorporating mindfulness can also enhance this balance. Mindfulness in sex means being present in the moment, fully engaging with the sensations and emotions that arise. As you explore G-Spot stimulation, take the time to check in with each other. Notice how your partner's body responds, and be attuned to subtle changes in their breathing or movements. This attentiveness fosters a deeper connection and turns the act into a shared experience rather than a solo pursuit of orgasm.

It's also important to recognize that every relationship will ebb and flow. There may be times when physical pleasure takes precedence and other times when emotional intimacy is more critical. The key is mutual respect and adaptability. If one partner feels that the balance is tipping too much in one direction, it's essential to address it gently and constructively. Periodic check-ins can help partners realign their sexual and emotional needs.

Lastly, it's vital to celebrate the small victories and milestones. Maybe you've discovered a new position that intensifies G-Spot stimulation, or you've learned something new about your partner's desires. These moments are worth cherishing. They not only enrich your sexual encounters but also strengthen your bond.

In summary, balancing pleasure and intimacy when integrating G-Spot stimulation into a healthy sex life is an ongoing dance. It's about nurturing emotional closeness while exploring physical pleasure, creating a symphony where both elements complement and enhance each other. Embrace the journey with an open heart and a curious mind, and you'll find that the blend of pleasure and intimacy will lead to a more fulfilled and connected partnership.

Holistic Approaches

Taking a holistic approach to integrating G-Spot stimulation into a healthy sex life means considering the whole person – their physical, emotional, and psychological well-being. It's not just about the mechanics but about creating a fulfilling and balanced intimate life that nurtures both partners. By being mindful of various aspects, one can foster a deeper connection and a more satisfying sexual experience.

Physical health forms a crucial foundation. Regular exercise, a balanced diet, and adequate sleep all contribute to one's overall energy levels and stamina, which can enhance sexual performance and enjoyment. Physical fitness isn't about achieving a specific body type but about maintaining a body that's capable and responsive. When your body feels good, you're more likely to feel confident and open to exploring new experiences, including G-Spot stimulation.

Emotional intimacy plays a significant role in holistic sexual experiences. Partners should focus on building trust and understanding through open communication. Talking about desires, boundaries, and preferences can remove the anxiety and insecurity often associated with sexual exploration. When both partners feel heard and valued, the emotional bond strengthens, paving the way for more profound physical connections.

It's also essential to recognize the mind-body connection. Stress, anxiety, and other mental health concerns can significantly impact one's sexual experience. Practices like mindfulness and meditation can help in staying present and engaged during intimate moments, allowing for a more authentic and pleasurable experience. Techniques such as deep breathing and body awareness can enhance the sensations associated with G-Spot stimulation, making it a more integrated experience.

Aromatherapy can serve as an adjunct to enhance the sensory experience. Scents like lavender, rose, and sandalwood are known for their relaxing properties and can create a soothing environment that makes exploration and connection more accessible. Utilizing diffusers, scented candles, or essential oils can help in establishing a calming, intimate space.

Beyond physical practices, fostering a supportive relationship environment is key. This includes being patient and empathetic towards each other's needs and vulnerabilities. Encouraging a non-judgmental space where both partners feel safe to express their inner fantasies and concerns can amplify the joy of discovery and mutual pleasure.

Spiritual practices can also be part of a holistic approach. For those who are spiritually inclined, rituals, prayers, or energy work can add a layer of depth to their intimate experiences. Practices like tantra that focus on the spiritual dimensions of sexuality can offer a pathway to exploring G-Spot stimulation in a way that transcends mere physical pleasure and enters the realm of the sublime.

Diet and nutrition can't be ignored either. Certain foods are known as aphrodisiacs and can enhance libido and energy levels. Incorporating foods rich in vitamins and minerals, such as zinc (found in oysters), antioxidants (abundant in berries), and omega-3 fatty acids (from fish like salmon) can elevate one's overall sexual health and vitality.

Regular check-ups and consultations with healthcare providers ensure that any underlying health issues that might impact sexual function are addressed. Conditions like hormonal imbalances or chronic illnesses should be managed appropriately, as they can affect sexual desire and responsiveness.

Incorporating holistic practices doesn't mean adhering to a rigid set of rules but rather integrating multiple facets of well-being to create a rich, fulfilling sex life. It's about understanding and honoring one's own body and emotions and being attuned to one's partner. Each of these components – physical health, emotional intimacy, mental mindfulness, and spiritual connection – interweave to form the tapestry of a thriving, joyful sexual relationship.

Ultimately, the goal is to create a space where both partners can explore and express their desires openly, feel supported, and find a deeper connection through their sexual experiences. Embracing a holistic approach can transform G-Spot stimulation from a mere physical act into a shared journey of discovery, trust, and love, enhancing not just sexual pleasure but also overall relationship satisfaction.

Knowing that each aspect of a person's well-being is integrated and that mindful practices can lead to heightened experiences, a holistic approach invites us to look beyond the surface and delve into a deeper, more connected way of enjoying our intimate lives.

Chapter 25:
Integrating P-Spot Stimulation
into a Healthy Sex Life

Integrating P-Spot stimulation into your sexual repertoire can be a transformative experience, heightening pleasure and deepening intimacy. It's about more than just discovering new sensations; it's about opening up communication with your partner, exploring vulnerability, and prioritizing mutual satisfaction. When embraced with curiosity and a spirit of shared journey, P-Spot stimulation can enrich your connection, making each encounter a discovery of both physical and emotional dimensions. Care, hygiene, and ongoing consent are key. Remember, sexual health is part of overall well-being, and integrating P-Spot play is another step in a loving and informed sexual relationship.

Combining Techniques

Integrating P-Spot stimulation into a healthy sex life opens up a realm of possibilities for maximizing sexual pleasure and connected intimacy. Combining techniques can amplify sensations and lead to profound levels of satisfaction, whether you're exploring alone or with a partner.

One of the first considerations is synchronization. Achieving harmony between different kinds of stimulation—such as blending P-Spot and penile techniques—can create waves of pleasure that build upon each other. Imagine stimulating the prostate while simultaneously engaging in penile stroking or oral pleasure. These dual actions can lead to mind-blowing orgasms and a deeper connection with your partner.

In solo play, combining techniques requires a keen sense of body awareness. Focus initially on the sensations brought about by one kind of stimulation, such as gentle massaging of the P-Spot with a finger or a toy. Once you're comfortable, start incorporating penile stimulation. Perhaps use your other hand or a second toy designed for penile pleasure. Alternating between P-Spot and penile focus can lead to a medley of sensations, ultimately heightening your sexual experience.

Adding different types of stimulation also allows for personalized experiences. No two individuals will respond to stimuli in exactly the same way. You might find the utmost pleasure in rhythmic P-Spot tapping combined with slow, deliberate strokes to the penis. Or maybe the magic lies in a continuous pressure on the prostate while receiving quicker, shallow penile movements. Discovering what works best for you is a journey in itself, one filled with discovery and excitement.

For couples, communication is paramount. Being open about preferences ensures both partners feel comfortable and engaged. Vocalizing what feels good or providing gentle guidance can transform the session from merely pleasurable to extraordinarily fulfilling. It's vital that both partners are attuned to each other's reactions. Small gestures or changes in breathing can indicate when it's time to intensify or ease up on stimulation.

Variation is another key strategy in combining techniques. Alternating between different kinds of touch and pressure keeps the experience dynamic and exhilarating. One moment could involve intense, focused P-Spot stimulation, while the next might shift to light, teasing touches on the penis. This variation prevents overstimulation and keeps the body in a constant state of delightful anticipation.

Using toys specifically designed for dual stimulation can be a game-changer. Some toys are engineered to stimulate the prostate internally while offering external vibration for the perineal area or penis, effectively bridging the gap between the two forms of pleasure. Whether vibrating prostate massagers or dildos with dual functionalities, incorporating these into your sexual routine can enhance the experience exponentially.

Incorporating breath and mindfulness into your routine can also amplify your sessions. Paying close attention to how your body responds, taking deep breaths, and focusing your mental energy on the sensations can heighten the experience. Mindfulness ensures you're fully present and receptive to every wave of pleasure, making the climax even more memorable.

For those venturing into combined techniques with a partner, trust is the cornerstone. A relationship built on open communication and mutual respect will enrich the sexual experience. Create an environment where talking about boundaries and limits feels normal, not awkward. This could mean agreeing on safe words or signals that either partner can use at any point.

Exploring P-Spot stimulation alongside other forms of pleasure doesn't always have to lead to orgasm as the sole goal. Sometimes, the journey can be just as fulfilling as the destination. Engage in sessions where the focus is purely on enjoying each other's bodies and the myriad sensations that come with varied stimulation techniques.

Another aspect worth considering is integrating lubricants. When combining techniques, adequate lubrication is essential for comfort and enhanced sensations. Opt for high-quality, body-safe lubes that don't dry out quickly. This simple addition can make the experience smoother and more enjoyable.

Setting the ambiance can be just as crucial. Dim lighting, soft music, and even scented candles can contribute to a relaxed and intimate atmosphere conducive to exploring dual-stimulation techniques. Feeling relaxed allows both partners to fully immerse themselves in the sensations without distractions, making the experience deeply intimate and gratifying.

Finding the perfect rhythm is like conducting an orchestra. The combination of P-Spot and penile stimulation requires a balanced cadence that ebbs and flows, bringing you or your partner closer to climax in waves rather than a quick spike. Listen to your bodies and let intuition guide you, adjusting pressure and speed as necessary.

When it comes to adding additional forms of touch, don't forget about the rest of the body. Incorporate elements like nipple stimulation, gentle caresses on the thighs, or even kisses and whispers. The synergy of these combined efforts can make the overall experience not just about the genitals but an all-encompassing, full-body sensation.

Ultimately, experimenting with combining techniques is a journey of exploration and discovery. It takes time, practice, and a willingness to communicate openly. But the rewards—a deeper connection with your partner and a more nuanced understanding of your own body—make every moment worth it.

Balance is key. Ensuring that the amount of time you spend on P-Spot stimulation is harmoniously offset by time spent on other areas of pleasure leads to a holistic sexual experience. It's this balance that makes the entire encounter feel less like a sequence of actions and more like a seamless, flowing dance.

Finding the right combination of techniques tailored to your unique preferences and incorporating them into your sexual routine requires patience and open-mindedness. But when done right, it can transform your sexual experiences into deeply fulfilling, multi-dimensional journeys of pleasure.

Maintaining a Healthy Sexual Relationship

Maintaining a healthy sexual relationship while integrating P-Spot stimulation is an art that combines communication, trust, and mutual respect. It's about creating a safe and loving environment where both partners feel valued and heard. Open communication is paramount. Discussing boundaries, preferences, and desires openly can transform the experience into something deeply intimate and mutually satisfying.

When beginning to explore P-Spot stimulation, it's crucial to start with a foundation of trust and understanding. Discussing expectations and concerns allows both partners to feel comfortable and respected. Trust isn't built overnight; it grows through consistent and honest communication. Expressing vulnerability and being supportive can strengthen the emotional and sexual bond between partners.

Variety plays a significant role in keeping intimacy alive. Exploring different techniques and experimenting with toys can introduce new sensations and keep the sexual relationship exciting. Remember, the focus should be on pleasure and enjoyment rather than achieving a goal. This mindset can alleviate pressure and make the experience more enjoyable for both partners.

One essential aspect of maintaining a healthy sexual relationship is prioritizing mutual pleasure. Ensuring both partners are equally invested in the experience enhances intimacy and connection. By focusing on each other's pleasure, you create a more balanced and satisfying relationship. Take time to understand your partner's cues and responses, and don't hesitate to ask questions. This ongoing dialogue fosters a deeper connection.

Incorporating P-Spot stimulation doesn't mean neglecting other forms of intimacy. Traditional acts like kissing, cuddling, and affectionate touch are integral to maintaining a healthy sexual relationship. These actions build a foundation of love and warmth that enhances the overall experience. Balancing P-Spot stimulation with other intimate practices ensures a well-rounded and fulfilling relationship.

Respect each other's boundaries and comfort levels. Not everyone may feel immediately comfortable with P-Spot exploration, and that's perfectly okay. Patience and understanding are key. Gradually introducing new elements and allowing time for adjustment can make the experience more comfortable and enjoyable. Always prioritize consent and ensure both partners are on the same page.

Routine isn't inherently bad, but mixing things up can significantly enhance your sexual life. Regularly trying new positions, settings, or techniques prevents the experience from becoming monotonous. This doesn't mean constant change; instead, it's about finding a rhythm that works for both partners while occasionally introducing new elements to keep things exciting.

Maintaining a healthy sexual relationship also involves taking care of your mental and physical well-being. A good diet, regular exercise, and stress management contribute to a more satisfying sexual experience. When both partners feel good about themselves, they're more likely to engage enthusiastically in sexual activities. Ensuring you're both in a healthy mental space can be just as important as physical readiness.

Emotional intimacy is as vital as physical intimacy. Sharing feelings, thoughts, and experiences strengthens the emotional connection and makes sexual experiences more profound. Spend quality time together outside the bedroom to build this emotional bond. Whether it's a shared hobby, a meaningful conversation, or simply enjoying each other's company, these moments contribute to a deeper connection.

Educational exploration can also foster a healthy sexual relationship. Couples who learn together about different techniques and body responses can better understand and satisfy each other. Reading books, attending workshops, or seeking advice from professionals can provide new insights and ideas. Knowledge empowers both partners to explore confidently and safely.

Another aspect to consider is the role of spontaneity and planned encounters. While spontaneity can add excitement, planned intimate moments ensure that both partners are ready and willing, thus enhancing the experience. Balancing these approaches keeps the relationship dynamic and enjoyable.

It's essential to recognize and celebrate each other's efforts. Complimentary feedback and encouragement can enhance self-esteem and make intimate experiences more rewarding. Affirming each other's desires and efforts creates a supportive and positive environment where both partners feel appreciated.

Maintaining a healthy sexual relationship while exploring new aspects like P-Spot stimulation requires a balanced approach. Focus on communication, trust, and mutual satisfaction to create a fulfilling and loving environment. By prioritizing these elements, couples can enhance their intimacy and build a resilient and pleasurable sexual relationship.

Conclusion

A s we reach the end of this journey through the fascinating realms of G-Spot and P-Spot stimulation, it's essential to reflect on the deeper insights we've uncovered. The intricacies of sexual pleasure, often shrouded in mystery and misunderstanding, have been laid bare through scientific research, personal exploration, and open communication. This isn't just a guide; it's an invitation to transform your intimate life.

Sexual pleasure, celebrated in countless cultures and histories, remains a deeply personal and transformative aspect of human experience. Understanding the anatomy and science behind the G-Spot and P-Spot provides a foundation, but it's the individualized exploration and emotional connection that breathe life into these concepts. This book has offered you the tools, techniques, and knowledge to embark on this exploration with confidence and curiosity.

The journey of discovering one's body and the bodies of our partners is as much about the mind as it is about physical sensations. The chapters delving into psychological aspects emphasize the profound connection between mental arousal and physical pleasure. Overcoming barriers—be they mental, emotional, or societal—is crucial for a fulfilling sexual experience. When approached with an open heart and mind, the process of learning and experimenting with different techniques can become a mutual journey of growth and discovery.

Communication stands as the bedrock of any intimate relationship. The chapters on partnered techniques and enhancing intimacy underscore the importance of dialogue—both verbal and non-verbal. Sharing your desires, boundaries, and experiences fosters a deeper bond and increases mutual satisfaction. Relationships thrive on this kind of open and empathetic communication, creating a safe space for continual exploration and joy.

Solo play, another crucial area covered, is often the first step towards self-discovery in sexual pleasure. Knowing your own body, what feels good, and how to achieve those magical sensations can be incredibly empowering. This self-understanding lays the groundwork for future exploration with partners, enabling clearer communication of wants and needs.

The advanced techniques laid out in the latter sections of the book are not just for seasoned enthusiasts but for anyone willing to push the envelope of their sexual experiences. They offer a pathway to intensifying pleasure, enhancing skills, and deepening intimate connections. Remember, sexual exploration is a lifelong journey, filled with endless possibilities and discoveries. There's always room for growth, no matter your level of experience.

Safety and hygiene, while perhaps not the most glamorous aspects of sexual exploration, are fundamentally important. Proper care and informed practices ensure that your experiences are not only pleasurable but also healthy and sustainable. By addressing common concerns and providing practical advice, this book aims to equip you with the knowledge to enjoy your exploration with peace of mind.

In tackling the myths and misconceptions surrounding the G-Spot and P-Spot, we aim to liberate you from false beliefs that might hinder your sexual potential. Dispelling these myths opens the door to a more honest, informed, and enriched sexual life. Knowledge dispels fear and replaces it with curiosity and confidence.

Our exploration would be incomplete without considering how these specific techniques integrate into a holistic sex life. Balance and integration are key. It's not about sidelining other aspects of intimacy but enriching the overall tapestry of your sexual relationship. The insights and techniques shared throughout this book are meant to be woven into the broader context of emotional intimacy, personal growth, and relational health.

At its core, this journey through G-Spot and P-Spot stimulation is about more than just physical pleasure. It's a path to deeper understanding and connection—to oneself and to one's partner. It's an invitation to live a more fully expressed and intimate life. As you continue to explore and apply the knowledge gained here, let curiosity be your guide and communication your ally.

Remember, your sexuality is an integral part of who you are, deserving of exploration, understanding, and celebration. Keep learning, keep experimenting, and most importantly, keep communicating. Through this ongoing journey, you have the potential to continually transform your sexual experiences into richer, more profound aspects of your life.

Thank you for embarking on this journey. Your commitment to understanding and enhancing sexual pleasure paves the way for a more intimate, satisfying, and joyous life. Embrace the discoveries you've made, and let them ignite the spark in your intimate relationships. Here's to a lifetime of pleasure, connection, and growth.

Appendix A:
Appendix

This section is dedicated to providing additional resources and supplementary information that will enhance your journey toward understanding and mastering G-Spot and P-Spot stimulation. The Appendix aims to offer practical advice, recommended readings, and tips that weren't covered in the main chapters, functioning as an extra layer of support for your ongoing exploration and learning.

Additional Tips for Enhancing Pleasure

While we've delved deeply into the techniques and science behind G-Spot and P-Spot stimulation, there are always more nuanced tips that can enrich your experience:

Mindfulness Practice: Incorporating mindfulness techniques can significantly deepen your sensual experiences. Being present in the moment and fully aware of your bodily sensations can heighten pleasure.

Breathing Exercises: Controlled breathing can play a pivotal role in sexual pleasure. Deep, rhythmic breathing can help you manage arousal levels and prolong your sexual experience.

Experiment with Props: Pillows and other soft supports can help you achieve and maintain optimal positions for G-Spot and P-Spot stimulation, thereby enhancing comfort and pleasure.

Recommended Products

In addition to the techniques covered in this book, various products can assist in making your exploration even more rewarding:

High-Quality Lubricants: Opt for lubricants free of harsh chemicals. Water-based options are generally safe and effective for most forms of stimulation.

Specialized Toys: There are countless toys designed specifically for G-Spot and P-Spot stimulation. Look for those with ergonomic shapes and customizable vibration settings to find what best suits your needs.

Relaxation Aids: Aromatherapy oils and calming music can create an inviting atmosphere, making it easier to relax and fully engage in the experience.

Journals and Tracking Progress

Keeping a journal can be a powerful tool in understanding your preferences and progress. Documenting your experiences can help you identify what techniques work best and how you can refine your approach over time.

Workshops and Courses

Numerous workshops and online courses are available for those looking to deepen their understanding further. These can provide hands-on experience and expert guidance, offering an invaluable complement to the information in this book.

Professional Guidance

If you encounter challenges or have specific concerns, consulting with a sex therapist or medical professional can provide personalized advice and support. Professional guidance can be instrumental in overcoming any mental or physical barriers you may face.

Building a Supportive Community

Engaging with supportive communities, whether online or in person, can offer encouragement and shared wisdom. Consider joining forums, attending meetups, or participating in social media groups focused on sexual health and pleasure.

Embrace this appendix as a continuing resource on your path to sexual enlightenment. Remember, this journey is unique to you, and every step you take is a testament to your commitment to building a richer, more fulfilling intimate life.

Glossary of Terms

This glossary aims to demystify and define the key terms and concepts you'll encounter as you journey through this book. Understanding these terms will empower you to navigate your intimate experiences with greater confidence and awareness.

Arousal: A physiological and psychological state of being that increases sexual desire and readiness for sexual activity.

Clitoris: A small, sensitive organ located at the top of the vulva, known for its significant role in female sexual pleasure.

Desensitization: A reduction in sensitivity, which can occur temporarily after prolonged or intense stimulation.

Erogenous Zones: Areas of the body that are particularly sensitive to touch and can elicit sexual arousal.

G-Spot: A sensitive area located within the anterior vaginal wall, known for its potential to enhance sexual pleasure and induce orgasms.

Lubrication: The natural or artificial substance that reduces friction during sexual activity, enhancing comfort and pleasure.

Mind-Body Connection: The interplay between mental and physical states, which can notably influence sexual experiences.

Orgasm: The peak of sexual pleasure characterized by intense physical and emotional sensations.

P-Spot: Also known as the prostate, a gland located near the male bladder, which can be stimulated to enhance sexual pleasure.

Prostate: A walnut-sized gland in males that can be stimulated for pleasure and is involved in the production of seminal fluid.

Refractory Period: The recovery phase after orgasm during which it is physiologically impossible for an individual to have another orgasm.

Stimulation: The act of arousing or increasing activity or interest in a sexual context, often through touch, movement, or devices.

Vagina: The muscular canal in females that extends from the vulva to the cervix, capable of significant expansion and sensitive to various forms of stimulation.

Vulva: The external part of the female genitalia, encompassing the labia, clitoris, and the opening of the vagina.

Definitions of Key Concepts

In order to fully appreciate and master G-Spot and P-Spot stimulation, it's essential to understand several key concepts that serve as the foundation for deeper exploration and enhanced pleasure. This section of the glossary aims to demystify these terms, providing clear and concise definitions that will help you navigate through the subsequent chapters with confidence and ease. From biological components to psychological principles, having a solid grasp of these concepts will allow you to apply various techniques more effectively and understand their impact on your intimate experiences.

G-Spot: The G-Spot, or Grafenberg Spot, is an area located within the anterior wall of the vagina, a few inches inside. Discovered by German gynecologist Ernst Gräfenberg, it is a sensitive region that, when stimulated correctly, can lead to intense pleasure and sometimes even ejaculation in individuals assigned female at birth (AFAB). Understanding its location and structure is crucial for both solo explorers and couples aiming to enhance their intimate moments.

P-Spot: The P-Spot, commonly referred to as the prostate, is a gland located just below the bladder in individuals assigned male at birth (AMAB). When stimulated, it can produce profound pleasurable sensations. It's not only essential for sexual performance but also plays a vital role in overall male sexual health. Knowing how to locate and stimulate the P-Spot can open up new dimensions of pleasure and satisfaction.

Stimulation Techniques: This term encompasses various methods used to stimulate the G-Spot and P-Spot to elicit sexual pleasure. Techniques can range from manual (using fingers) to advanced (incorporating sex toys) methods. Each technique has unique benefits and challenges, and understanding these can significantly enhance one's ability to achieve and give pleasure.

Solo Play: Solo play refers to the act of sexually pleasuring oneself. In the context of this book, it involves techniques for G-Spot and P-Spot stimulation that individuals can practice on their own. Solo play is an essential part of sexual well-being as it allows individuals to understand their bodies better, identify what feels good, and explore new ways of experiencing pleasure.

Couples Play: Couples play involves the integration of G-Spot and P-Spot stimulation techniques within the dynamics of a relationship. It involves mutual exploration, communication, and understanding to enhance intimacy and sexual satisfaction. Couples play not only deepens physical connection but also strengthens the emotional bond between partners.

Sexual Response Cycle: This concept, delineated by Masters and Johnson, is a four-phase process that describes the sequence of physical and emotional changes that occur as a person becomes sexually aroused and participates in sexually stimulating activities. The phases include excitement, plateau, orgasm, and resolution. Understanding this cycle can help in recognizing how G-Spot and P-Spot stimulation fits into broader sexual experiences.

Mind-Body Connection: The intricate relationship between one's mental state and physical responses during sexual activities. This connection plays a pivotal role in G-Spot and P-Spot stimulation, as mental preparedness and a relaxed state of mind can significantly enhance physical pleasure. Recognizing the importance of a healthy mindset allows for more meaningful and satisfying experiences.

Sexual Health: This broad term encompasses the overall well-being related to sexuality. It includes physical health, such as the functioning of sexual organs and systems, as well as mental and emotional states, such as feeling comfortable and confident about one's sexuality. Practicing safe and hygienic techniques for G-Spot and P-Spot stimulation is crucial for maintaining sexual health.

Communication: Open and honest dialogue about sexual preferences, boundaries, and experiences is vital for both solo and partnered play. Effective communication ensures that all participants are comfortable, consensual, and fully enjoying the experience. It also helps in exploring new techniques and eliminating misunderstandings related to G-Spot and P-Spot exploration.

Safety and Hygiene: These terms refer to the best practices and precautions necessary to prevent infections, injuries, and other health issues during G-Spot and P-Spot stimulation. Safety and hygiene include using clean and appropriate toys, washing hands, and understanding the body's reactions to different types of stimuli.

Blended Orgasms: An orgasm resulting from the simultaneous stimulation of multiple erogenous zones, such as the G-Spot and the clitoris or the P-Spot and the penis. Blended orgasms can lead to more intense and satisfying sexual experiences. Understanding and mastering the techniques for achieving blended orgasms can elevate the quality of sexual pleasure.

Myths and Misconceptions: Throughout the book, you'll encounter various myths and misconceptions about G-Spot and P-Spot stimulation. These are incorrect beliefs or ideas that may hinder the understanding and exploration of sexual pleasure. Dispelling these myths with factual, scientific information helps in creating a more accurate and positive approach to sexual health.

Emotional Preparedness: Being emotionally ready involves understanding and managing feelings of vulnerability, excitement, and anticipation that come with exploring new facets of sexual pleasure. It's particularly important in P-Spot and G-Spot stimulation, as these involve intimate areas that require a high level of trust and comfort, especially in partnered scenarios.

Sexual Pleasure: A complex, multi-dimensional experience that involves physical sensations, emotional connections, and psychological states. The aim of mastering G-Spot and P-Spot stimulation techniques is to enrich the overall spectrum of sexual pleasure, making it a more fulfilling and profound experience. Being well-versed in these key concepts allows for a holistic understanding and practical application, ensuring that the journey toward enhanced intimacy is both enlightening and pleasurable.

As we journey through the intricate world of G-Spot and P-Spot stimulation, these key concepts will serve as your guideposts. Comprehending these definitions ensures a well-rounded approach, enabling you to seamlessly integrate new knowledge and techniques into your intimate life. Exploring these foundational ideas not only empowers you but also enhances the joy and connection you share with your partner or yourself, making every moment of exploration truly enriching.

Understanding Technical Terms

In any domain of expertise, understanding specific technical terms is crucial to mastery and confidence. When it comes to sexual pleasure and intimate activities, there exist a multitude of terms and phrases that can appear intimidating or confusing at first. By demystifying these terms, we can empower both individuals and couples to feel knowledgeable and assured in their explorations.

Sexual anatomy is a fundamental aspect that requires clear understanding. The G-Spot, for example, is not merely a vague concept but a distinct area within the female anatomy that, when stimulated, can result in powerful sensations and orgasms. Similarly, the P-Spot—often referred to as the prostate—plays a vital role in male sexual pleasure. It's essential to understand these terms not just as anatomical references but as components of a broader sexual framework.

Another particularly important term is "erogenous zone." These are sensitive areas on the body that tend to respond positively to touch and can facilitate arousal. While some zones are well-known, such as the nipples or the inner thighs, others are less discussed but equally significant. Knowing where these zones are and how they can contribute to sexual pleasure helps in making informed and intentional decisions during intimate moments.

The concept of "sexual response cycle" is another key term that aids in understanding how our bodies react during different stages of arousal and climax. This cycle typically includes phases like excitement, plateau, orgasm, and resolution. Recognizing these stages can help individuals and couples identify where they might want to focus their energies and how to prolong or enhance certain experiences.

"Stimulation" is a term you'll frequently come across, particularly in a guide focused on enhancing pleasure. This involves applying various forms of touch or pressure to different parts of the body to elicit pleasure. Techniques for stimulation can vary drastically, from gentle caresses to more intense forms of interaction, and understanding these variations can help in tailoring experiences to individual preferences.

In the realm of tools and toys, terms such as "vibrator," "dildo," and "anal beads" need to be well-understood. Each of these tools has a specific function and design tailored to stimulate either the G-Spot, P-Spot, or other erogenous zones. Familiarity with these terms allows readers to choose the right tool for their needs and use them effectively.

One shouldn't overlook the importance of "lubrication" in these discussions. Natural lubrication can be complemented with artificial lubricants to ensure comfort and safety during intimate activities. Different types of lubricants, such as water-based, silicone-based, and oil-based, offer various benefits and potential drawbacks. Knowing when and how to use each type can vastly enhance the experience and prevent discomfort.

"Consent" is perhaps one of the most crucial terms in the glossary of sexual pleasure. An understanding of consent is vital for any healthy sexual relationship. It involves clear, informed, and voluntary agreement to engage in a specific activity. In the context of exploring new types of sexual stimulation, ongoing consent and open communication are fundamental to ensuring a positive and respectful experience for all parties involved.

Then there are psychological terms like "arousal," "desire," and "libido." These terms explain the mental and emotional aspects of sexual pleasure. Understanding them can provide significant insights into how mental states can influence physical sensations and vice versa. Recognizing the complex interplay between mind and body can be revolutionary in achieving deeper, more fulfilling experiences.

Just as important are the clinical terms often encountered in scientific research. Terms like "neurotransmitters" and "hormones" play a critical role in understanding the biological mechanics behind sexual pleasure. These chemicals, such as oxytocin and dopamine, can profoundly influence our sensations and emotional responses during intimate moments.

"Safety" and "hygiene" are also terms that frequently appear in discussions about sexual pleasure techniques. Safety involves understanding the limits of one's body, knowing how to avoid injuries, and recognizing when something feels off. Hygiene revolves around practices such as cleaning toys and hands, which are essential to prevent infections and maintain a healthy sex life.

Taking the time to grasp these technical terms adds a layer of understanding and respect to the conversations around sexual pleasure. It transforms these discussions from taboo or uncomfortable topics into empowering, informed dialogues. By knowing the language of this intimate domain, individuals and couples can communicate more effectively, explore more confidently, and enjoy more profoundly.

Overall, understanding these technical terms equips you to dive deeper into the complex, beautiful, and incredibly rewarding realm of sexual pleasure. It's about creating a shared vocabulary that not only bridges gaps in knowledge but also strengthens connections. Having this foundation allows for exploration with a sense of curiosity and confidence, making every intimate experience not just more enjoyable but profoundly enriching.

Chapter 26:
Further Reading and Resources

In your journey to deepen your understanding of sexual pleasure, it's essential to seek out varied perspectives and continually enrich your knowledge. This chapter offers a curated selection of recommended books, articles, and online resources that delve further into G-Spot and P-Spot stimulation, providing valuable insights and advanced techniques. From scientific studies to expert advice, you will find resources that cater to both solo explorers and couples eager to enhance their intimate connections. Engaging with these materials will not only empower you with information but also inspire you to confidently navigate your personal pleasure map and foster deeper intimacy with your partner. Embrace the opportunity to learn from the best minds in sexual health and intimacy, and transform your understanding into a more fulfilling and adventurous sensual experience.

Recommended Books and Articles

In your journey to deepen your understanding of sexual pleasure, insightful literature and academic research can be indispensable. A wealth of knowledge exists that can enhance your intimate experiences through G-Spot and P-Spot stimulation. The following books and articles have been carefully curated to expand your perspectives and equip you with advanced knowledge.

"Come As You Are" by Emily Nagoski: This book delves deep into the science of sex and sexuality, presenting informative and relatable content. Nagoski's evidence-based approach deciphers underlying mechanisms of sexual response and offers practical advice to better understand and enhance sexual pleasure.

"Mating in Captivity" by Esther Perel: Renowned for her insights into the intricacies of desire and intimacy, Perel's work explores how couples can reconcile the need for security and the pursuit of passion. Although not solely focused on G-Spot or P-Spot stimulation, her discussions on enhancing intimacy can serve as a foundation for successful exploration in these areas.

"The Hite Report" by Shere Hite: A pioneering work in the study of female sexuality, this seminal report collects first-hand accounts and statistical data to paint a comprehensive picture of women's sexual experiences. Understanding the diversity of sexual pleasure can be instrumental in recognizing and appreciating the individual nuances of G-Spot and P-Spot stimulation.

"Anal Pleasure & Health" by Jack Morin: This book is a thorough, research-backed guide to understanding anal pleasure and health. Morin's compassionate and informative writing breaks taboos and provides a solid foundation for exploring P-Spot stimulation safely and pleasurably.

"She Comes First" by Ian Kerner: Kerner's work is highly focused on the importance of female pleasure in heterosexual relationships. By emphasizing techniques and strategies specifically for the G-Spot, Kerner provides actionable advice that aligns well with enhancing G-Spot stimulation.

"The Multi-Orgasmic Man" by Mantak Chia and Douglas Abrams: Exploring the full spectrum of male sexuality and techniques for achieving multiple orgasms, this book touches upon the importance of the P-Spot. It provides a holistic view on enhancing male sexual health and pleasure.

Beyond these books, several articles and academic papers provide a more technical perspective on G-Spot and P-Spot anatomy and stimulation:

"The G-Spot Phenomenon: A Clinical Study" by Ernst Gräfenberg: As a landmark study, Gräfenberg's work introduced the concept of the G-Spot, laying a foundation for further investigation into female sexual pleasure.

"Anatomy and Physiology of Sexual Function in Men" by Irwin Goldstein: This work delves into the intricacies of male sexual anatomy, including the prostate, providing essential insights that can be directly applied to P-Spot stimulation techniques.

"Sexual Response Cycles and Their Implications" by William Masters and Virginia Johnson: Their thorough exploration of human sexual response cycles is vital for understanding the context within which G-Spot and P-Spot stimulation occur.

Additionally, these articles and studies help bridge the gap between practical techniques and theoretical knowledge:

"Neurobiology of Sexual Pleasure: The Role of the Brain" by Barry Komisaruk: This in-depth article examines how different brain regions are involved in sexual response, elucidating the neural underpinnings of G-Spot and P-Spot stimulation.

"The Prostate as an Organ of Sexual Function: A Review" by John P. Mulhall: Mulhall's review compiles key scientific findings about the prostate's dual role in reproduction and pleasure, offering valuable understanding for P-Spot exploration.

"Clinical Perspectives on the G-Spot" by Beverly Whipple: Whipple's work synthesizes clinical findings and personal narratives to map out a

clear guide to the realities and misconceptions surrounding the G-Spot.

If you prefer reading more recent articles, consider exploring online academic journals like The Journal of Sexual Medicine or The International Journal of Impotence Research. These journals often feature the latest studies and findings that can keep you updated on cutting-edge research:

"Exploring the Influence of Partner Dynamics on Sexual Satisfaction" by Janice Y. Marks: Found in The Journal of Sexual Medicine, this article investigates how relationship factors affect sexual pleasure, touching upon the role of communication in fostering effective G-Spot and P-Spot stimulation.

"Sexual Function and Health: A Review of Clinical Studies" by Marcia D. Kennedy: Published in The International Journal of Impotence Research, this comprehensive review covers a range of studies related to both G-Spot and P-Spot stimulation, offering a robust reference for deeper understanding.

To truly appreciate the depth of sexual pleasure and its many facets, engaging with these books and articles can provide both relational and scientific perspectives. Each resource contributes a unique piece to the complex puzzle of sexual intimacy, helping to build a well-rounded, informed approach to G-Spot and P-Spot stimulation. While the above recommendations serve as a solid starting point, the field of sexual health continually evolves, prompting the importance of staying curious and updated with ongoing research.

Finally, don't hesitate to explore the plethora of forums and discussions within online communities dedicated to sexual health and pleasure. Websites like Reddit's r/sex and specialized forums provide anecdotal experiences and community advice, often reflecting a diversity of perspectives and approaches that can enhance your personal explorations and understanding.

Empower yourself with knowledge, be open to new findings, and remember that the path to sexual pleasure is as much about journeying with curiosity as it is about the destination itself.

Online Resources and Communities

The journey toward understanding and enhancing intimate pleasure doesn't have to be a solitary one. With the rise of the internet, an enormous wealth of information and supportive communities have become accessible at the click of a button. These digital spaces offer a platform for individuals and couples to learn, share experiences, and grow in their understanding of sexual wellness. This section delves into the various online resources and communities that can guide and inspire your exploration of G-Spot and P-Spot stimulation.

One of the most valuable online resources is educational websites and blogs dedicated to sexual health and wellness. Websites such as *Scarleteen* and *GoAskAlice* provide medically reviewed content and practical advice on a broad range of topics, including anatomical exploration and stimulation techniques. These platforms offer not just information but also a sense of community and belonging, helping readers feel less isolated in their curiosity and experiences.

Another vital resource is online forums and discussion boards. Websites like *Reddit* host numerous subreddits such as *r/Sex* and *r/sexualhealth*, where users can openly ask questions, share personal experiences, and seek advice from a global community. These forums are often moderated to ensure respectful and informative discussions, making them a safe space for exploring intimate topics that may be difficult to bring up in face-to-face conversations.

Social media platforms also play a significant role in fostering communities around sexual pleasure and health. Instagram accounts run by sex educators, such as @sexwithdrjess and @shanboody, disseminate bite-sized, accessible information. These accounts frequently address questions from followers and create content that is both educational and engaging. Similarly, YouTube channels hosted by sex therapists and educators provide in-depth discussions and visual demonstrations that can be incredibly informative.

Online workshops and webinars present another excellent opportunity to deepen your understanding. Many sex educators and therapists offer virtual classes covering a wide array of topics, from the basics of sexual anatomy to advanced techniques for achieving blended orgasms. These sessions often include interactive components, allowing participants to ask questions and receive personalized advice in real-time. Websites like *OMGS* and *Babeland* frequently host such events, providing a structured yet flexible learning environment.

For those looking to dive deeper into academic and clinical perspectives on sexual health, online databases and journals are invaluable. Websites like *PubMed* and *Google Scholar* offer access to peer-reviewed studies and articles that can provide a more scientific understanding of G-Spot and P-Spot stimulation. These platforms are especially useful for those who appreciate evidence-based information and wish to stay updated on the latest research findings in the field.

Podcasts also serve as an excellent resource for those who prefer auditory learning. Shows like *"Sex with Emily"* and *"The Pleasure Mechanics"* cover a vast array of topics related to sexual pleasure and health, often featuring expert guests who provide unique insights and practical tips. Podcasts offer a convenient way to absorb information while on the go, making it easier to integrate learning into a busy lifestyle.

For individuals and couples interested in a more personalized approach, online counseling and therapy services can be incredibly beneficial. Platforms such as *Talkspace* and *BetterHelp* connect users with licensed therapists specializing in sexual health and relationships. These services provide a confidential environment to discuss personal concerns, challenges, and goals, offering professional guidance tailored to your specific needs.

Moreover, the importance of community support in exploring sexual pleasure cannot be overstated. Online support groups and communities dedicated to specific aspects of sexual health provide a venue for mutual support and encouragement. Facebook groups, for instance, offer closed or secret groups focusing on various interests, from exploring new techniques to coping with sexual dysfunctions. These communities often build strong bonds among members, creating a sense of belonging and shared purpose.

Online retailers specializing in sexual wellness products, such as *Lovehoney* and *Sh!*, also offer a wealth of information through user reviews and detailed product descriptions. These platforms frequently feature expert advice and how-to guides that can aid in selecting the right products for G-Spot and P-Spot stimulation, ensuring a safer and more pleasurable experience.

Finally, eBooks and digital guides provide a treasure trove of information, often delving into topics with a level of detail and depth that other online resources may not match. Many respected sex educators and therapists publish their work digitally, making it easy to download and read at your own pace. Platforms like *Amazon Kindle* and *Apple Books* offer extensive libraries dedicated to sexual health and pleasure, ensuring that you have access to authoritative, insightful content whenever you need it.

As you embark on this journey of exploration and discovery, remember that the digital landscape is rich with resources and communities eager to support you. Whether you're seeking technical guidance, emotional support, or a community of like-minded individuals, the internet has something to offer. Harness the collective wisdom and experiences available online to enhance your intimate life and deepen your understanding of sexual pleasure.

Ultimately, the digital world is a gateway to endless possibilities. By leveraging these online resources and communities, you can cultivate a fulfilling and knowledgeable approach to G-Spot and P-Spot stimulation, enriching both your solo and shared experiences. Don't hesitate to explore, ask questions, and connect with others on this exciting journey towards greater sexual wellness and pleasure.

www.ingramcontent.com/pod-product-compliance
Lightning Source LLC
Chambersburg PA
CBHW030321290526
45785CB00001B/456